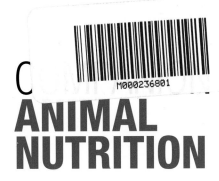

C

ANIMAL
NUTRITION

For Elsevier:

Commissioning Editor: Rita Demetriou-Swanwick
Development Editor: Louisa Welch
Project Manager: Elouise Ball
Designer: Charles Gray
Illustration Manager: Bruce Hogarth, Gillian Richards
Illustrator: Samantha Elmhurst

COMPANION ANIMAL NUTRITION

Nicola Ackerman BSc Hons VN C&GCertSAN

Senior Medical Nurse,
The Veterinary Hospital Group,
Estover, Plymouth, UK

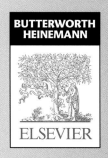

Edinburgh   London   New York   Oxford   Philadelphia   St Louis   Sydney   Toronto   2008

BUTTERWORTH
HEINEMANN
ELSEVIER

First published 2008

ISBN: 978-0-7506-8898-7

British Library Cataloguing in Publication Data
A catalogue record for this book is available from the British Library

Library of Congress Cataloging in Publication Data
A catalog record for this book is available from the Library of Congress

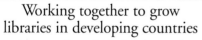

Working together to grow
libraries in developing countries

www.elsevier.com | www.bookaid.org | www.sabre.org

ELSEVIER   BOOK AID
International   Sabre Foundation

your source for books,
journals and multimedia
in the health sciences

www.elsevierhealth.com

The
publisher's
policy is to use
**paper manufactured
from sustainable forests**

Printed in China

Contents

Preface

The role of nutrition in both medical and surgical cases has greatly improved the well-being and longevity of patients. No longer is the goal of nutrition just to prevent deficiencies. The use of nutrition in a holistic approach to patient care should not be an afterthought, but an integral aspect of any nursing care plan, in both long-term chronic and short-term acute cases. All patients should be treated as individuals, and the nutritional status of each needs to be assessed prior to deciding on a specific diet or nutritional regimen.

Advising on an appropriate diet is only one stage in establishing and promoting well-being. Providing information on transferring onto a new diet, and, if any side effects occur, providing the owner with any support or advice, make nutrition a long-term involvement requiring input from the veterinary practice. As disease processes advance or in some cases improve, changes in nutritional support are required, whilst in healthy animals, correct nutrition throughout life for the appropriate life-stage, breed and work levels is required.

This text hopes to cover the most commonly experienced medical conditions, feeding pre- and postoperatively, and the feeding of healthy animals. Case studies will be used to demonstrate how individual cases respond to different nutrients, and thus affect the diet of choice.

Over 90% of exotic animals presented to veterinary practices have husbandry-related diseases or disorders. Client education is paramount in preventing ill health and behavioural problems, and improving longevity. Nutrition plays a major role in these factors, and support to these owners must be provided, along with literature that they can take home, read and digest.

Many commercial dietary manufacturers do provide expert veterinary advice on individual cases and useful websites, and should be utilized in obtaining guidance. Literature provided by these companies can also prove to be beneficial and informative for clients. Access to a named nurse or technician if difficulties arise should be promoted, as a holistic approach can only be achieved if all the elements of the care plan are implemented. Additional educational development for the nurse, technician, or veterinary surgeon concerning nutrition, should always be promoted within the veterinary practice.

This text is aimed at anyone who wishes to enhance the quality of life of veterinary patients in a holistic approach with the use of nutrition.

Nicola Ackerman,
2008

Acknowledgements

A huge thank you must go to Christopher and Ellena Ackerman, and to our parents, for their love and support throughout the procedure of researching and writing of the book.

I would also like to thank the Veterinary Hospital Group in Plymouth for aiding in providing case studies, radiographs and photographs.

Lastly, I would like to thank Rita Demetriou-Swanwick at Elsevier, for all of her help.

List of Abbreviations

AAFCO	Association of American Feed Control Officials
ACE	Angiotensin-converting enzyme
ALKP	Alkaline phosphatase
ALT	Alanine aminotransferase
ARD	Antibiotic responsive diarrhoea
AST	Aspartate aminotransferase
ATP	Adenosine triphosphate
BCS	Body condition score
BEE	Basal energy expenditure
BER	Basal energy requirement
BMR	Basal metabolic rate
BUN	Blood urea nitrogen
BV	Biological value
BW(kg)	Bodyweight (in kilograms)
CK	Creatine kinase
COPD	Chronic obstructive pulmonary disease
CP	Crude protein
CRF	Chronic renal failure
CS	Chondroitin sulphate
D+	Diarrhoea
DCM	Dilated cardiomyopathy
DCP	Dyschondroplasia
DE	Digestible energy
DER	Daily energy requirement
DHA	Docosahexaenoic acid
DMB	Dry matter base
DOD	Developmental orthopaedic disease
EAA	Essential amino acids
EFA	Essential fatty acids
EMS	Equine metabolic syndrome
EPA	Eicosapentaenoic acid
EPI	Exocrine pancreatic insufficiency
ER	Exertional rhabdomyolysis
FAD	Flea allergic dermatitis
FLUTD	Feline lower urinary tract disease
GAG	Glycoaminoglycans
GDV	Gastric dilation/volvulus
GE	Gross energy
GI(T)	Gastrointestinal (tract)
HE	Hepatic encephalopathy
HI	Heat increment
IBD	Inflammatory bowel disease
IBS	Irritable bowel syndrome
IDDM	Insulin-dependent diabetes mellitus
MBD	Metabolic bone disorder
MCS	Muscle condition score
MCT	Medium-chained triglycerides
ME	Metabolizable energy
MER	Maintenance energy requirements
MMP	Matrix metalloproteinases
NE	Net energy
NFE	Nitrogen-free extract
NIDDM	Non-insulin-dependent diabetes mellitus
NRC	National Research Council
NSAID	Non-steroidal anti-inflammatory drug
OA	Osteoarthritis
OCD	Osteochondritis dissecans
PEG	Percutaneous endoscopic gastrostomy
PEM	Protein energy malnutrition
PLGE	Protein-losing gastroenteropathy
PN	Parenteral nutrition
POTZ	Preferred optimum temperature zone
PPN	Partial/peripheral parenteral nutrition
PSS	Portal systemic shunts
PUFA	Polyunsaturated fatty acids
RAA	Renin–angiotensin–aldosterone
RAO	Recurrent airway obstruction
RER	Resting energy requirements
ROS	Reactive oxygen species
SAMe	S-Adenosylmethionine
SCFA	Short-chain fatty acid
SH	Sodium hyluranate

SIBO	Small intestinal bacterial overgrowth	**TPR**	Temperature, pulse and respiration
TB	Thoroughbred	**UV**	Ultraviolet
TCA	Tricarboxylic acid	**V+**	Vomiting
TLI	Trypsin-like immunoreactivity	**VFA**	Volatile fatty acid
TPN	Total parenteral nutrition	**VLDL**	Very low-density lipoprotein

section 1

Anatomy and Physiology

1

Anatomy and physiology of the digestive system

The digestive system is required to ingest, digest, absorb, metabolize and excrete materials that have been obtained for utilization of required nutrients. The digestive system (Fig. 1.1) consists of:

- Oral cavity (lips, tongue and teeth)
- Pharynx
- Oesophagus
- Stomach
- Small intestine (comprising duodenum, jejunum and ileum)
- Large intestine (caecum, colon, rectum and anus)
- Accessory organs (salivary glands, pancreas, gall bladder (in cats and dogs) and the liver).

Oral cavity

The oral, or buccal cavity contains the teeth, tongue and salivary ducts. The cavity is formed by the incisive bone and maxilla forming the upper jaw, the palatine bone (hard palate) and the mandible forming the lower jaw. The functions of the oral cavity include:

- *Prehension.* The lips and tongue are used to pick up or obtain the food. The use of the lips in this process is essential in rabbits and horses.
- *Mastication.* Mastication or chewing is used to break down the food into small boluses prior to swallowing.
- *Lubrication.* The bolus of food is mixed with saliva in order to make swallowing easier.
- *Digestion.* Digestion of some carbohydrates starts within the oral cavity. This process does not

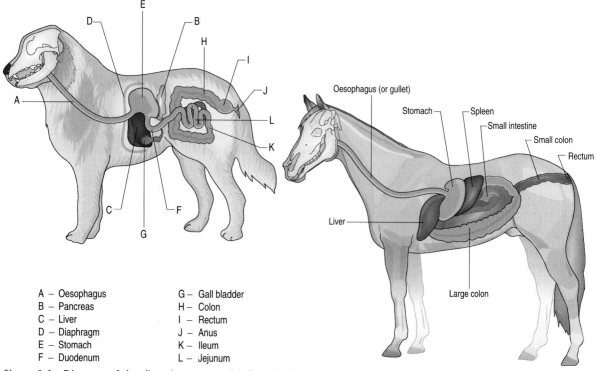

A – Oesophagus   G – Gall bladder
B – Pancreas   H – Colon
C – Liver   I – Rectum
D – Diaphragm   J – Anus
E – Stomach   K – Ileum
F – Duodenum   L – Jejunum

Figure 1.1 Diagram of the digestive system: (a) dog; (b) horse.

occur in carnivores like cats and dogs. This is due to the limited period of time that the food remains within the mouth.[1]

Teeth

There are two basic types of teeth in mammals, brachyodont and hypsodont. Brachyodont teeth are present in cats and dogs, and have a short crown-to-root ratio, and a true root. The hypsodont tooth, present in rabbits, horses, guinea pigs and chinchillas, has a long crown and a comparatively short root. These teeth are either radicular or aradicular. Horses have radicular teeth and they eventually form a true root. Rabbits, guinea pigs and chinchillas have aradicular hypsodont teeth;[2] these teeth never form a true root with an apex and the tooth grows continuously throughout the animal's life. This continuous growth is necessary due to the continual grinding of vegetation during mastication. Problems arise when this process is prevented, and are further discussed in Chapter 9 (p. 87).

Rabbit formula:

2 × {I2/1 : C0/0 : P3/2 : M3/3}

Dog formulae:

Primary teeth 2 × {Di3/3 : Dc1/1 : Dp3/3} = 28

Permanent teeth 2 × {I3/3 : C1/1 : P4/4 : M2/3} = 42

Cat formulae:

Primary teeth 2 × {Di3/3 : Dc1/1 : Dp3/2} = 26

Permanent teeth 2 × {I3/3 : C1/1 : P3/2 : M1/1} = 30

Horse formulae:

Primary teeth 2 × (Di3/3 : Dc0/0 : Dp3/3) = 24

Permanent teeth 2 × (I3/3 : C1/1 : P3 or 4/3 : M3/3) = 40 or 42

The action of the teeth is to tear, shred and grind the consumed diet. The tongue helps mix the food with saliva and forms the mixture into a bolus, which is pushed by the tongue into the pharynx and swallowed. By means of peristalsis, the bolus moves down the oesophagus into the stomach. The cardiac sphincter marks the entrance to the stomach, and relaxes when the pressure from the food bolus builds up behind it.

Salivary glands

The salivary glands are situated in pairs around the oral cavity. The saliva, a mixture of 99% water and 1% mucus, enters the cavity via salivary ducts. In omnivores and herbivores the saliva also contains enzymes. The salivary glands are made up of the zygomatic, sublingual, mandibular and parotid glands. Apart from its function in lubricating the food bolus and enzymatic breakdown (in some species), saliva is also used in thermoregulation. Evaporation of saliva from the tongue (in panting), or hair when applied during grooming helps to cool the animal. In equines, saliva is continuously secreted, and up to 10–12 l per day can be produced in a normally fed horse.[3]

Stomach

The stomach lies on the left side of the cranial abdomen. The function of the stomach is to act as a reservoir for the food, to break up the food (mechanical digestion), and to begin the process of protein digestion (chemical digestion). The stomach is able to accommodate the volume of food consumed because of deep longitudinal folds within its wall, called rugae. The rugae flatten out as the stomach fills with food. Distension of the stomach stimulates the secretion of gastrin. Gastrin initiates the production of the gastric juices.

The stomach can be divided into three regions, the cardia, fundus and pylorus, with most of the gastric glands being situated within the fundic region (the main body of the stomach). The gastric mucosa (lining of the stomach) contains the gastric pits, which consist of three types of cells that secrete the gastric juices, the goblet, parietal and chief cells (Table 1.1).

Once food has been broken up and mixed with the gastric juices the mixture is called chyme. The stomach via the pyloric sphincter releases chyme at intervals into the duodenum. This is dependent on the type of food consumed. Foods high in fat will remain in the stomach for longer periods of time, as digestion takes longer. When the stomach is empty 'whole organ' contractions occur. This causes emptying of all swallowed saliva, gastric secretions or refluxed intestinal secretions back into the duodenum. These specific contractions are referred to as housekeeper contractions.

Rhythmic segmentation occurs in the stomach and through to the large intestines. Rhythmic segmentation is vital in ensuring that chyme is adequately mixed, and that absorption of nutrients can occur thoroughly. If this process did not occur only the nutrients on the outside of the chyme bolus would come in contact with the intestinal lumen and be absorbed.

Small intestine

The small intestine is made up of the duodenum, jejunum and ileum. Chyme passes through the small intestine by means of peristalsis and rhythmic segmentation. The duodenum is in a fixed position because of the short mesentery. The pancreatic duct and common bile duct enter into the duodenum. Intrinsic glands (those within the intestinal wall) such as Brunner's glands secrete digestive

Table 1.1 Component and function of secretions produced by the cells within the gastric mucosa

Cell type	Gastric juice component	Function
Goblet cell	Mucus	Lubrication, protects gastric mucosa from autodigestion
Parietal cell	Hydrochloric acid (HCl)	Denatures proteins by creating an acidic environment of pH 1.3–5
Chief cell	Pepsinogen	The HCl converts pepsinogen to pepsin, which hydrolyses proteins into peptides

enzymes. It is within this initial third of the small intestine that the main portion of mammalian enzymatic digestion occurs. The main nutrient absorption occurs within the lumen of the jejunum and ileum. The intestinal juices are produced by Brunner's glands in the duodenum (these secretions are known as *succus entericus*), and crypts of Lieberkühn in the jejunum and ileum. The epithelial layer of the small intestine is folded into villi (Fig. 1.2). The function of this folding is to increase the total surface area and increase absorption and digestion. This surface area is further increased by microvilli on the villi, creating a brush border.

Pancreas

The pancreas is a mixed organ, possessing endo- and exocrine functions. In the process of digestion, the exocrine portion of the organ is required. The pancreas secretes pancreatic enzymes and bicarbonate, which make up the pancreatic juices (Table 1.2). The juices are secreted into the duodenum via the pancreatic duct.

Large intestine

The large intestine is made up of the caecum, colon, rectum and anal sphincter (anus). The caecum joins the small intestine at the ileocaecal junction. In carnivores the caecum serves no significant function, but in hindgut fermenters the caecum plays a highly significant role. Mammals are unable to digest cellulose, but the microflora within the caecum ferments the fibre into short-chain fatty acids (SCFA)/volatile fatty acids (VFA), which the animal uses as an energy source.

The ileocaecal valve divides the small and large intestine. This can be the site of parasitic burdens, especially of tapeworms in equines. The caecum is a vestigial organ in the cat, of moderate size in the dog, and voluminous and sacculated in the horse and rabbit.[4] In rabbits and equines the caecum acts as a fermentation chamber. Microbial flora breaks down the cellulose plant cell walls and proteins into VFA. The VFA are absorbed into the circulation through capillaries in the caecal epithelium.[5]

In the rabbit this semi-liquid material passes through to the colon where the solid, fibrous and indigestible particles are separated out through colon contractions. This material is then passed as hard faeces. The softer, non-fibrous material is passed back into the caecum to undergo further fermentation, through retropulsive contractions. This material is excreted as caecotrophs, often at night. These green caecotrophs are rich in protein, the vitamins B and K, and VFA. The rabbit will usually consume the caecotrophs directly from the anus. Generally the

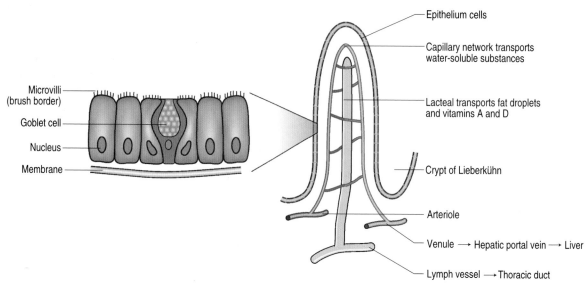

Figure 1.2 Diagram of an intestinal villus.

Table 1.2 Function of the components of the pancreatic juices

Component of pancreatic juices	Function
Bicarbonate	Neutralizes gastric acid in order to gain an optimal pH for pancreatic enzymes to work
Trypsinogen	Converted to trypsin by enterokinase
Lipase	Activated by bile salts, converts lipids into glycerol and fatty acids
Amylase	Breaks down carbohydrates to maltose
Maltase	Converts maltose to glucose
Sucrase	Converts sucrose to glucose and fructose
Lactase	Converts lactose to glucose and galactose
Enterokinase	Converts trypsinogen to trypsin
Aminopeptidase	Breaks down peptides to amino acids

caecotrophs are covered in thick mucus. This is to protect them as they pass through the stomach into the small intestine, where the nutrients can be absorbed.

The colon is divided into the ascending, transverse and descending colon, which relates to its position within the abdominal cavity. The function of the colon is to absorb water, water-soluble vitamins and electrolytes.

The rectum is classed as the part of the colon running through the pelvic cavity to the anal sphincter. The function of the rectum is to store faeces prior to defecation. The anal sphincter is made up of two muscular rings, the internal and external sphincters, which control the process of defecation. The lumens of the two sphincters are lined with longitudinal folds in order to allow for the passage of faeces. The internal sphincter is under involuntary control, whereas the external sphincter is controlled voluntarily.

The anal glands (modified sebaceous glands) in cats and dogs are situated between the two anal sphincters. Animals fed on softer, low-fibre diets can have the potential to have difficulties in emptying the glands sufficiently enough. Impaction of the glands can result; in these cases a diet with an increased fibre content is recommended.

The liver

The liver is the largest organ in the body, and plays a significant role in digestion and metabolism of nutrients.

1. *Carbohydrate metabolism.* The pancreas is responsible for the production of insulin, which allows glucose to enter the cells from the bloodstream. Excess glucose is converted to glycogen by glycogenesis in the liver. The reverse process (glycogenolysis) occurs when the blood glucose levels become low.

2. *Protein metabolism.* The liver has several roles involving protein metabolism. These include production of the plasma proteins albumin, fibrinogen, prothrombin and globulin, and regulation of amino acids in the processes of transamination and deamination.

3. *Fat metabolism.* The liver converts fatty acids and glycerol into phospholipids and to cholesterol for bile salts.

4. *Formation of bile.* Bile is stored in the gall bladder in some species (e.g. cats and dogs); in herbivores, bile is released into the intestinal tract constantly because of differences in feeding habits.

5. *Storage of vitamins,* especially the fat-soluble vitamins (A, D, E and K), but also some of the water-soluble vitamins.

6. *Storage of iron.* Most of this iron is temporary and comes from the breakdown of old erythrocytes; it is stored for later use in the manufacture of new erythrocytes in the bone marrow.

Other functions of the liver not related to digestion include formation of red blood cells in the fetus, storage of blood, breakdown of haemoglobin, hormone production and breakdown, regulation of body temperature and production of heat, and the detoxification of harmful substances.

Endocrine system

The inclusion of the endocrine system within a nutrition text is mandatory. Interactions of hormones with nutrient intake play a large role in vitamin, mineral and energy utilization and storage. Understanding of the physiology of the endocrine system is required, especially that of the homeostasis of calcium and phosphorus and glucose levels, when discussing clinical nutrition.

Calcium and phosphorus homeostasis

Secretion of parathormone from the parathyroid glands is dependent on the blood calcium levels. When blood calcium levels become low, calcium is resorbed from the bones and absorption from the intestine is increased (Fig. 1.3). Care should be taken when diagnosing hypocalcaemia, as blood calcium levels can be normal, due to calcium resorption from bones occurring, leading to a false positive result. Ionized calcium levels should be monitored and requested when submitting blood samples to look at hypocalcaemia. In dogs, a correct calcium level can be calculated to account for this, by use of this formula:[6]

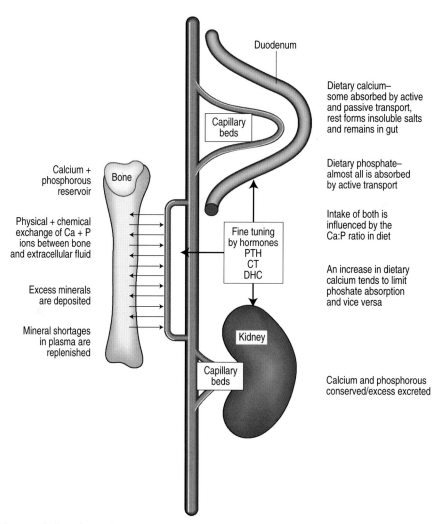

Duodenum

Dietary calcium– some absorbed by active and passive transport, rest forms insoluble salts and remains in gut

Capillary beds

Calcium + phosphorous reservoir

Bone

Dietary phosphate– almost all is absorbed by active transport

Physical + chemical exchange of Ca + P ions between bone and extracellular fluid

Fine tuning by hormones PTH CT DHC

Intake of both is influenced by the Ca:P ratio in diet

An increase in dietary calcium tends to limit phoshate absorption and vice versa

Excess minerals are deposited

Mineral shortages in plasma are replenished

Kidney

Capillary beds

Calcium and phosphorous conserved/excess excreted

Figure 1.3 Calcium and phosphorus homeostasis.

Correct calcium level (mmol/l) = [{Measured calcium (mmol/l) × 4} – {Albumin (g/dl)/10} + 3.5] × 0.25

Hyperparathyroidism can occur in three different ways:

1. *Primary hyperparathyroidism* is caused through direct disease to the parathyroid glands, i.e. neoplasia. Clinical signs include bone resorption, bone weakness and pathological fractures.

2. *Secondary hyperparathyroidism* is seen as a result of chronic renal failure. As the renal function becomes impaired the ratio of calcium to phosphorus in the blood becomes altered. The consequence of this is an increased secretion of parathormone and thus an increased resorption of calcium from bones in order to maintain homeostasis of calcium levels. With secondary hyperparathyroidism there is a preferred resorption of calcium from the jawbones (mandible and maxilla); this produces the condition referred to as 'rubber jaw'.

3. *Nutritional hyperparathyroidism* results from a nutritional deficiency of calcium in the diet. This is commonly seen in all meat diets, which also have high levels of phosphorus, and bran diets.

Glucose homeostasis

The pancreas, a mixed gland, controls homeostasis of blood glucose levels. The islets of Langerhans secrete three hormones that regulate blood glucose levels. The interactions of these hormones aid in obtaining homeostasis throughout the day, as food is consumed and energy utilized.

1. *Insulin (from the beta cells)*. When the blood glucose levels increase as a response to eating, insulin is released. The action of insulin is to lower the blood glucose levels by enabling cells to take up glucose and thus utilize it as a source of energy, and by storing excess glucose as glycogen in the liver. This process is known as glycogenesis.

2. *Glucagon (from the alpha cells)*. When blood glucose levels are low, glucagon is released. This hormone stimulates the breakdown of glycogen to glucose (glycogenolysis) in the liver.

3. *Somatostatin (from the alpha cells)*. This hormone is a mild inhibitor of the secretion of insulin and glucagons. This aids in preventing large fluctuations in blood glucose levels.

Diabetes mellitus results from a failure of the animal to produce insulin. This can be as a result of a number of reasons, which are discussed in full in a later section. The role of nutrition is paramount in this condition, as are the routines surrounding feeding (diet, timing and quantities) and daily exercise levels. When trying to stabilize patients suffering from diabetes mellitus, over-swings can occur in response to other hormones.

Absorption of nutrients

Nutrients are absorbed throughout the intestine and by a number of different means.

■ *Osmosis or passive transport*. This process occurs when a solute moves from an area of high concentration to one of low concentration. This process is not actively used, because once the level of the nutrient in the bloodstream reaches the same concentration as the intestinal lumen osmosis will stop as a state of equilibrium has been achieved.

■ *Active transport*. This process is the main way in which carbohydrates and proteins are absorbed. Active transport occurs across cell membranes with the use of adenosine triphosphate (ATP). This process is advantageous as it is not dependent on concentration gradients.

The absorption and digestion of fats occurs in a more complex manner. Triglycerides present within the diet are emulsified by bile salts within the duodenum. The enzyme lipase is activated by the presence of the bile salts and breaks the triglycerides down into glycerol and fatty acids. Once emulsified and in this state they are referred to as micelles. The micelles are absorbed into the mucosal cells where triglyceride resynthesis occurs and chylomicron production occurs. The chylomicrons are absorbed through the walls of the intestinal villi into the lacteals. The milky liquid that is formed is chyle, and is transported through the lacteals to the cisterna chyli before entering the circulation via the thoracic duct (Fig. 1.4).

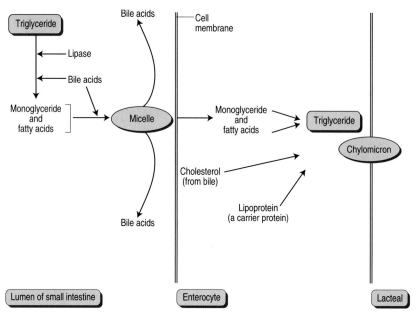

Figure 1.4   Diagrammatic representation of fat absorption.

References

1. Aspinall V, O'Reilly M. Introduction to veterinary anatomy and physiology. Edinburgh: Butterworth-Heinemann; 2004.
2. Gorrel C, Derbyshire S. Veterinary dentistry for the nurse and technician. Edinburgh: Elsevier Butterworth-Heinemann; 2005.
3. Frape DF. Equine nutrition and feeding. 2nd edn. Oxford: Blackwell Science; 1998.
4. Maskell IE, Johnson JV. Digestion and absorption. In: Burger I, ed. The Waltham book of companion animal nutrition. Oxford: Pergamon Press; 1993:25–44.
5. Aspinall V. Anatomy and physiology: Part 3 – The rabbit. VN Times 2005; (Dec):11–12.
6. Gough A. Calcium disorders of dogs and cats: Part 1 Calcium pathophysiology. UK Vet 2004; 9(5):32–33.

section 2

Nutrients and Digestion

2
Nutrients

In order to design or implement a diet for a particular lifestage or clinical problem, understanding of nutrient requirements and availability, and consequences of deficiencies or excesses, is important. Nutrients are divided into six basic categories:

- Water
- Proteins
- Lipids (fats, oils and waxes)
- Carbohydrates
- Vitamins
- Minerals.

Water

Water is the most vital of all nutrients, and assessment of hydration levels of all animals should be performed (Box 2.1). When clinically examining an animal, assessing water intake and giving advice to owners on how animals can increase intake is beneficial (Appendix 4).

Functions

Water has several important functions within the body. It is required:

- as the solvent in which substances such as soluble materials (vitamins and hormones) and waste products (urea) are dissolved and transported around the body
- in chemical reactions that involve hydrolysis, such as the catabolism of other nutrients
- in thermoregulation, via the evaporation of water from the tongue (in panting) or skin (in sweating); large amounts of energy are required to evaporate small amounts of water, thus conserving water supplies
- as a lubricant for body tissues, e.g. pleural surfactant and synovial fluids
- as a major component of blood and lymph, creating a medium for these cells to be circulated in.
- as a major constituent of milk
- as protection (e.g. embryonic fluids).

Requirements

Body water is lost through urination, defecation, cutaneous and respiratory routes. Respiratory and cutaneous losses are referred to as inevitable losses as the animal has no control over them. Water is either derived from metabolic processes or con-

sumed as a liquid or as part of the diet. The daily water requirements of a dog, cat or horse are estimated at 50–60 ml/kg bodyweight (BW)/day, and in dogs and cats are roughly equivalent to the daily energy requirements (DER) in kcal/day.[1] Consumption of a moist diet will lead to a decrease in consumption in liquid amounts. Daily water consumption can be greatly increased during lactation, and if activity levels increase dramatically. Clinical illness can cause polyuria, and thus polydipsia.

Deficiencies

Dehydration in the animal always needs to be corrected before any nutritional requirements are met. Haemoconcentration will greatly alter any blood biochemistries or haematology performed, and can be used to assess levels of hydration and any changes over a short period of time. Table 2.1 shows clinical signs associated with dehydration.

Excesses

Excesses of water are removed via urination; daily output should be 1–2 ml/kg BW/hour. Water should never be limited unless prior to anaesthesia or during deprivation testing. Excesses, via overinfusion or clinical disease, can lead to pulmonary effusion,

Table 2.1 Assessing levels of dehydration in an animal

Percentage of dehydration	Clinical signs
< 5%	No obvious outward signs Concentrated urine
5–8%	Slightly prolonged CRT Slight tenting of the skin Mucous membranes feel tacky Third eyelid visible
8–10%	Sunken eyes Prolonged CRT Obvious tenting of the skin
10–12%	Oliguria Tented skin remains in place Clinical shock can be experienced
> 12%	Progressive shock Coma and death

CRT, capillary refill time

oedema or ascites. Polydipsia can result in polyuria and a resulting loss in water-soluble substances, i.e. vitamins.

Carbohydrates

Carbohydrates range from simple sugars to dietary fibre. All carbohydrates have the general formula $(CH_2O)_n$ and use hydrolysis when being broken down into mono- or disaccharides. Carbohydrates can be subdivided into:

- monosaccharides, simple sugars (e.g. glucose)
- disaccharides, two sugars bonded together with the loss of one molecule of water, e.g.

> glucose + glucose = maltose
>
> glucose + fructose = sucrose

- oligosaccharides, three to nine sugar units, e.g. raffinose and stachyose
- polysaccharides, more than nine sugar units, e.g. amylose, amylopectin and glycogen.

Polysaccharides are complex sugars, and the nature of the bonding between the sugar units has a dramatic effect on digestion. Mammalian enzymes such as amylase can only break alpha bonds; only microbial enzymes can break beta bonds. Starches are made up of straight glucose chains of alpha 1,4 bonds (amylose) and with alpha 1,6 bonds that form branches. Starch found within plants is called amylopectin, yet within animals, starches are called glycogen. Fibre is an example of a polysaccharide, and has an important function in the diet, so much so that it will be discussed separately.

Functions

Carbohydrates are not essential within the diet, as other nutrients (amino acids and glycerol) can be used as precursors of glucose. The presence of carbohydrates within the diet does spare these precursors for their essential functions. The functions of carbohydrates include:

- As an energy source. Energy is provided (adenosine triphosphate; ATP) via glycolysis and the tricarboxylic acid (TCA) cycle (Fig. 2.1).
- Can be metabolized for energy to carbon dioxide and water, with the production of heat.

- Once metabolized can be used as building blocks for other nutrients such as non-essential amino acids, glycoproteins, glycolipids, lactose (important during lactation) and vitamin C.
- Can be stored as glycogen or converted and stored as fat.

Requirements

The daily nutritional requirements for carbohydrates are dependent on the energy requirements of the individual animal. During periods of high energy demands or when new tissue growth is occurring (e.g. growth, gestation or lactation), carbohydrates can be said to be conditionally essential in order to maintain these metabolic processes.

Deficiencies

Deficiencies in dietary carbohydrates place strain on other metabolic pathways such as lipid and protein in order to supply glucose precursors. If the provision of adequate glucose is met through these pathways, this can remove these precursors from body protein synthesis requirements. Cats have a unique metabolism and can maintain adequate blood glucose levels on a low-carbohydrate, high-protein diet.

Excesses

An excess of dietary carbohydrates can lead to weight gain, as glucose is converted to fat. Because of the previously mentioned metabolic differences between cats and dogs, excessive quantities of carbohydrates in cats can lead to maldigestion (diarrhoea and bloating), and adverse metabolic effects (hyperglycaemia and a consequent glucosuria). Persistent hyperglycaemia can lead to glucose intolerance and/or insulin resistance. Insulin resistance laminitis can be induced in horses; this can be attributed to a carbohydrate overload.

Fibre

Fibre is a complex carbohydrate, but its functions and requirements are different from those of the simple sugars and starches. Fibre differs from starch in that fibre resists digestion by mammalian enzymes. Digestion occurs in the colon in dogs

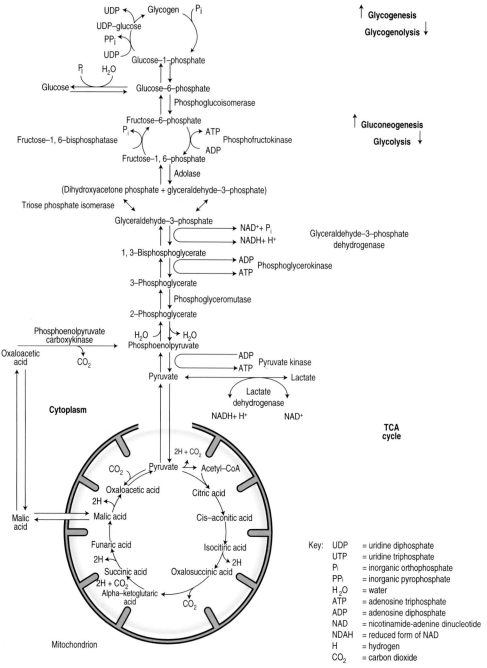

Figure 2.1 Biochemical pathways of glycogenesis, glycogenolysis, gluconeogenesis, glycolysis and the TCA cycle.

and cats, and the caecum in horses and rabbits, by microbes. This process, when utilized in rabbits and horses, is regarded as hindgut fermentation; evolutionary adaptation of the caecum has occurred in order to accommodate this process. Fibres include cellulose, hemicellulose, pectin, gums and resistant starches. Fibre can be subdivided according to its solubility in water:

Soluble – pectin, fructans, galactans

Insoluble – cellulose, hemicellulose, lignin

or biologically according to its utilization by intestinal bacteria:

Rapidly fermentable – fructans, galactans, guar gum

Moderately fermentable – pectin, beet pulp

Slowly fermentable – cellulose.

Functions

Fibre is not classified as a nutrient, but its inclusion within the diet can be highly beneficial for digestive health. Fibre affects functioning of the gastrointestinal tract by:

- delaying gastric emptying
- altering nutrient absorption and metabolism (can be both advantageous and disadvantageous)
- normalizing gastrointestinal transit time
- aiding maintenance of the structural integrity of the gastrointestinal mucosa
- increasing bulk and water in the intestinal contents
- decreasing overall digestibility of the diet.

Requirements

Fibre is not considered as an essential component of the diet, and individual requirements differ depending on lifestage and clinical requirements. In healthy animals a small amount of fibre (less than 5%)[2] that contains both soluble and insoluble fibres is recommended. In herbivores the recommendation of larger amounts of fibre is required. Effects of dietary fibre on physiological function within the animal are detailed in Table 2.2.

Deficiencies

Fibre deficiencies are not commonly noted in cats or dogs. However, deficiencies in the hindgut fermenters, rabbits and horses, can be very damaging. Low levels of fibre can result in dental problems and diarrhoea (especially in rabbits). In cats and dogs small amounts of dietary fibre are recommended as it produces the short-chain fatty acids (SCFA)/volatile fatty acids (VFA) which the intestinal microbes use as an energy source.

Excesses

Excess amounts of fibre can cause binding of required nutrients such as minerals. If deficiencies in certain minerals have been identified, consideration should be made of dietary fibre levels.

Proteins

Proteins consist of polypeptide chains of amino acids. There are 23 naturally occurring amino acids, which can be bonded into an infinite variety of proteins.

Proteins are able to combine with non-protein sources (e.g. iron) to form conjugated proteins (e.g. haemoglobin). Amino acids can be divided into two groups: essential and non-essential. Essential amino acids are those that cannot be synthesized within the body, and must be obtained from the diet. Some amino acids such as cystine and tyrosine can be described as conditionally essential. They are only essential when the diet is deficient in methionine and phenylalanine. The ten essential amino acids in the dog are:

Table 2.2 Effects of fibre on the physiological functioning of animals

Physiological function	Soluble/fermentable fibre	Insoluble/non-fermentable fibre
Gastric emptying	Decreased	Some increase
Pancreatic secretion	No effect	No effect
Nutrient absorption	No effect	No effect
Small intestinal transit	Decreased	Increased
Large intestinal transit	Decreased	Increased
Intestinal mucosal; mass	Increased	No effect
Microbial growth	Increased	No effect
Toxin binding	No effect	Increased

arginine, histidine, isoleucine, leucine, lysine, methionine, phenylalanine, threonine, tryptophan and valine.

The cat requires the same ten amino acids plus taurine.

The quality or biological value (BV) of proteins is the quantity of that protein which is utilized by the animals. The BV can be expressed as a percentage or as a decimal, and can be applied to all nutrients (carbohydrate, fatty acids), but is primarily used for proteins. A high-quality protein that has a high BV will contain all or most of the essential amino acids. Egg has a BV of 100%, cereals a BV of ~40–50%, dependent on soil grown in and type of cereals. Table 2.3 demonstrates some biological values of certain food types.

Commercial food labels do not describe the level of BV of the contained proteins, only the percentage of protein as fed, or dry matter base (DMB). Confusion can occur when interpreting quantity of dietary levels of proteins rather than quality of the proteins. Detailed analysis of the BV of the ingredients is also required.

Functions
- Proteins are primarily used as structural components of body organs and tissues, including:
  - collagen and elastin, present in the soft tissues of the musculoskeletal system
  - the contractile proteins actin and myosin, used in muscle contraction
  - keratin proteins, within skin, hair and nails
  - blood proteins, including haemoglobin, albumin and globulin.
- Proteins function as enzymes, hormones and antibodies.

Table 2.3 Biological values of certain foodstuffs

| Food | Biological value | |
	As percentage	As decimal
Egg	100	1
Milk	92	0.92
Meat	78 (variable)	0.78
Wheat	48 (variable)	0.48

- They are used as an energy source, after the process of deamination.
- They are used as the nitrogen source, for further production of DNA and other nitrogen-containing substances.

Requirements
The body is in a constant state of regeneration and flux, and the requirement for protein is constant. It can be increased during phases of growth, gestation and lactation, but also when there are inadequate supplies of carbohydrates for energy. Illness and tissue regeneration will also increase requirements; burns and scalds require larger amounts of protein than any other factor. Protein requirements for an adult dog and cat on a DMB are 18% and 26% respectively, puppies and kittens 22% and 30%, based on the Association of American Feed Control Officials' (AAFCO) recommendations.[2] This is based on a diet with commonly available protein sources. If the protein fed is of a high quality these values can be decreased, demonstrating the importance of using high-quality proteins in low-protein diets. The requirements in diets specifically for different diseases are discussed in detail in later sections.

Deficiencies
Initial deficiencies in protein can cause the clinical signs of reduced growth rate, poor coat and skin, anaemia, alopecia, reduction in fertility and reduced milk production during lactation. If protein deficiencies continue, a reduction in the lean body mass will occur, resulting in muscle atrophy and reduction in blood levels of albumin and other blood proteins.

Excesses
Protein or amino acid toxicity is not a practical problem in healthy animals, due to the deamination processes. High protein levels can cause problems in diseased animals, especially those with liver or kidney disease, where the deamination and removal of waste products is impaired. High-protein diets can also prove to be problematic when struvite dissolution is required or when adverse food reactions occur within the animal. Additional protein (over and above recommended amounts) in the diet does not have any positive effects. Excessive amounts are converted (deamination) to energy sources. Diets

aimed at adult maintenance should not exceed 30% (DMB) in dogs and 45% (DMB) in cats.[2]

Lipids

Lipids are made up of fats (which are solid at room temperature), oils (liquid at room temperature) and waxes. Lipids can be subdivided into single lipids and conjugated lipids. The single lipids include short-, medium- and long-chain fatty acids and esters of fatty acids with glycerol. Of these single lipids, triglycerides are the most commonly found in food. Conjugated lipids are lipids which have combined with other products, e.g. phospholipids (used in cell membranes).

Fatty acids with the first double bond between the third and fourth carbon belong to the n-3 group; when the bond is between the sixth and seventh carbon they belong to the n-6 group. The n-3 and n-6 fatty acids are the essential fatty acids (EFA), as animals cannot synthesize them themselves. EFA in the dog and cat include linolenic (n-3) and linoleic acid (n-6); arachidonic acid (n-6) is also essential in the cat. Adult dogs are able to synthesize linolenic and arachidonic acid from linoleic acid. Adult cats, however, can synthesize linolenic acid but not arachidonic acid. Arachidonic acid is only found in fat sources from animals, another reason why cats are obligate carnivores. Other important n-3 fatty acids include eicosapentaenoic (EPA) and docosahexaenoic (DHA) acids.

Functions
Lipids have many functions, which include:

- Meeting energy requirements – on a weight basis, dietary fat is approximately 2.25 times more energy dense than proteins and carbohydrates. When stored as adipose tissue, the quantity of energy available per gram is double that of carbohydrates.
- Absorption of the fat-soluble vitamins A, D, E and K.
- Phospholipids are required for structural support (e.g. cell membranes).
- Protection of internal organs by fat pads.
- Insulation, especially important in certain mammals in cold climates.

- Hormones, e.g. aldosterone and prostaglandins.
- Manufacture of eicosanoids.
- Waterproofing of fur and feather.
- Improving the palatability of foods.

Requirements
The absolute requirement for lipids is for an adequate supply of the essential fatty acids (EFA). Use of lipids as an energy supply can be exceptionally beneficial, especially in animals with high energy requirements. Increased fat utilization occurs during aerobic exercise.

Deficiencies
Deficiencies in lipids can cause a dry coat and scaly skin. A reduction of lipids on the skin can cause a predisposition to pyoderma. Wound healing can also be impaired due to the requirement of phospholipids within cell membranes. If there is a chronic deficiency of lipids, especially of the EFA, symptoms of alopecia, oedema and moist dermatitis can occur. Severe deficiencies can result in emaciation of the animal.

Excesses
Increased quantities of lipids within the diet directly relates to an increase in the energy density of the diet. Excess fat is stored as adipose tissue in the tissues and around the internal organs. Obesity can arise if excess energy intake to expenditure occurs. Excess fats within the diet can predispose the animal to pancreatitis and hyperlipidaemia.

Vitamins

Vitamins are organic compounds that are essential in small amounts for normal physiological functioning of the body. Not all vitamins are essential in all species, for example vitamin C is essential for guinea pigs, but not for cats and dogs. Vitamins can be described as fat-soluble or water-soluble. The fat-soluble vitamins (A, D, E and K) are absorbed from the gastrointestinal tract with fats, and are stored alongside the fat within the body. Daily intake is not always required because of the quantities stored and intestinal microbial production (Table 2.4). The water-soluble vitamins (B complex and C) are

Table 2.4   The function of fat-soluble vitamins, and consequences of deficiencies and toxicities

Vitamin	Function	Source	Deficiencies	Toxicity
Vitamin A (retinol)	Component of the visual pigments in the eye. Involved in cell differentiation and maintenance of cell structure	Liver, cod liver oil, kidneys and egg yolk	Night blindness, infertility, crusting lesions of the nares, seborrhoeic coat conditions, increased susceptibility to microbial infections	Liver damage, ankylosis of the joints, particularly cervical vertebrae and the long bones of the forelimbs
Vitamin D	Stimulates calcium absorption from the intestine. Participates in resorption of calcium from the bones	Can be synthesized from lipid compounds in the skin following exposure to UV light. Can be consumed preformed from the diet in fish oils, egg yolk and dairy products	Rickets in the young, and osteomalacia in adults	Can result in hypercalcaemia, which if prolonged results in extensive calcification of the soft tissues, lungs, kidneys and stomach. Deforms the teeth and jaw
Vitamin E	Protects cell membranes against oxidative damage	Liver, fats, and wheat germ	Pansteatitis (yellow fat disease). Skeletal muscle dystrophy, reproductive failure and impairment of the immune response in dogs	Very unlikely to occur, because relatively high doses are well tolerated
Vitamin K	Regulates the formation of clotting factors, (factors VII, IX, X and XII)	Bacterial synthesis in the intestine. Also found in green vegetables	Unlikely to occur owing to synthesis of the vitamin by intestinal bacteria, unless a vitamin K antagonist (warfarin) has been consumed, causing haemorrhaging	Can cause anaemia and other blood abnormalities in young animals

absorbed via the gastrointestinal tract, but can be lost in the urine. Supplementation of these vitamins may be required when polyuria is present (Table 2.5).

Minerals

A mineral is the term used to describe all the inorganic substances and elements (including salts) within the body and diet. These substances consti-

tute the ash component of the diet and make up less than 1% of total bodyweight. Minerals can be divided into three subgroups based on amounts required by the body.

Macrominerals

Macrominerals are expressed as parts per hundred (pph), with 1 pph = 10 g/kg diet. Their functions, sources, deficiencies and excesses are described in Table 2.6.

Table 2.5 The function of water-soluble vitamins, and consequences of deficiencies and toxicities

Vitamin	Function	Source	Deficiency	Toxicity
Vitamin B$_1$ (thiamin)	Involved in carbohydrate metabolism and maintenance of the nervous system	Yeast, fish, egg yolks, cereals and green vegetables	Anorexia, neurological disorders. Can be induced if large amounts of raw fish are fed – it contains the enzyme thiaminase	Thiamin has a low toxicity
Vitamin B$_2$ (riboflavin)	Essential for cellular growth, carbohydrate, fat and protein metabolism and correct growth	Liver, kidneys, milk, eggs and cereals. Some synthesis in the intestines	Lesions of the eyes, skin disorders and testicular hypoplasia	Not reported
Pantothenic acid	A constituent of coenzyme A, essential for carbohydrate, fat and amino acid metabolism	Liver, kidneys, eggs and wheat germ	Fatty liver, gastrointestinal disturbances, convulsions, depressed growth	Not reported
Niacin (nicotinamide and nicotinic acid)	A component of two coenzymes, which are required for oxidation–reduction reactions necessary for the utilization of all major nutrients	Meats, liver, fish, rice, potatoes, pulses	Can cause 'blacktongue' in cats and dogs	Not considered toxic
Vitamin B$_6$ (pyridoxine)	Involved in numerous enzyme systems that are associated with nitrogen and amino acid metabolism	Muscle meats, eggs, cereals and vegetables	Anorexia, weight loss and anaemia	Not considered toxic
Biotin	Aids in maintaining the integrity of keratinized structures (hair and nails). Also required for metabolism of fats and amino acids	Bacterial synthesis within the intestines. Dietary source can be from liver, kidneys, egg yolk, milk and yeast	Dry, scaly skin, brittle hair, hyperkeratosis, pruritus and skin ulcers. Unlikely to occur owing to bacterial synthesis, but care should be taken after periods of antibiotic use, or if raw egg whites, which contain avidin, are fed	Not reported
Folic acid	Maturation of red blood cells within the bone marrow. Nucleic acid synthesis and cell replication	Fish, liver, kidneys, yeast, also synthesized within the intestines	Anaemia and leucopenia, but deficiency unlikely because of intestinal bacterial synthesis	Not reported
Vitamin B$_{12}$ (cyanocobalamin)	Function closely linked to that of folic acid. Also involved in fat and carbohydrate metabolism	Liver, kidneys and heart	Pernicious anaemia and neurological signs	Not reported

Cont'd

Table 2.5 Cont'd

Vitamin	Function	Source	Deficiency	Toxicity
Vitamin C (ascorbic acid)	Wound healing, capillary and mucosal integrity	Normally synthesized from glucose. Guinea pigs and humans need to obtain it from the diet (fresh fruit and vegetables)	Scurvy	Not reported

Microminerals

Microminerals are expressed as parts per million (ppm), with 1 ppm = 1 mg/kg diet. Their functions, sources, deficiencies and excesses are described in Table 2.7.

Trace elements

These minerals act as catalysts at a cellular level; the amounts required in the diet are not yet known. It is thought that the quantities would be expressed as µg/kg diet. Examples of trace elements include chromium, cobalt, fluorine, molybdenum, nickel, silicon, sulphur and vanadium.

Antioxidants

The use of antioxidants in the diet is becoming more widely recognized as a positive influence in the health of animals and humans (Table 2.8). Antioxidants are used to neutralize the ill effects of free radicals (reactive oxygen species; ROS) within the body. Free radicals are produced as by-products of chemical reactions necessary to sustain life, e.g. cellular respiration. Damage caused is dependent on the balance between the antioxidants and free radicals within the body. The influence of free radical scavengers (vitamins E and C, carotenoids and selenium) is significant, and plays a role in the ageing process, contributing to the development and/or exacerbation of a wide variety of degenerative disease. There are many factors that can contribute to excessive levels of free radicals being produced. These include exposure to UV light and radiation, air pollution (including cigarette smoke), residues from herbicides and pesticides, and illness and the medications used to treat it. In some illnesses

patients in human medicine are actively encouraged to take antioxidants; these include sufferers of diabetes mellitus, arthritis and cancers. Owing to improved medical care, nutrition and veterinary guidance, animals are living longer. The incidence of cognitive dysfunction is increasing, and the use of nutrition in these cases has proved to be beneficial (see p. 129).

The use of antioxidants in equine nutrition should also be advocated. Examples where antioxidant use is beneficial include:

- Horses in training, as the body steps up to combat increased free radical production from exercise.
- Horses with recurrent airway obstruction (RAO)/chronic obstructive pulmonary disease (COPD) respond positively to antioxidant supplementation.
- Horses receiving oil are more likely to have free radicals due to polyunsaturated carbon bonds. Liquid perioxides form and cause further free radical damage.

Pre- and probiotics

Prebiotics are substances that are able to alter the gastrointestinal flora in a manner to benefit the microorganisms. Probiotics, however, are a live microbial feed supplement, which benefits the host animal by improving the gastrointestinal microbial population. Probiotics generally used comprise lactic acid bacteria such as lactobacilli, streptococci and bifidobacteria. Probiotics have been shown to be beneficial following acute gastroenteritis or a course of antibiotics, especially in hindgut fermenters such as rabbits and horses. Live yoghurt has similar beneficial effects; the

Table 2.6 The function and source of macrominerals, and consequences of deficiencies and excesses

Macromineral	Function	Source	Deficiency	Toxicity
Calcium (Ca)	Maintaining structural rigidity of bones and teeth, blood clotting, muscle and nerve function and enzyme activation	Milk, eggs, green vegetables	Nutritional secondary hyperparathyroidism. In lactating bitches hypocalcaemia results in eclampsia. Nervous disturbances	Conditions relating to excessive calcium intake during growth include hip dysplasia, osteo-chondrosis, and wobbler syndrome
Chloride (Cl⁻)	Maintenance of osmotic pressure, acid–base and water balance. Major component of bile and hydrochloric acid (gastric juices)	Common salt	Inability to maintain water balance, retarded growth, exhaustion, fatigue	Greater than normal fluid intake and consequently polyuria
Magnesium (Mg)	Required for healthy teeth and bones, energy metabolism and enzyme activation	Meat and green vegetables	Muscular weakness	With very high intakes there is an association with an increased incidence of feline lower urinary tract disease (FLUTD)
Phosphorus (P)	Development of teeth and bones, energy utilization, phospholipids in cell membranes, constituent of nucleic acids	Milk, eggs, meat, vegetables		If calcium levels are correspondingly low, ratio of calcium to phosphorus is imbalanced and hypocalcaemia is induced
Potassium (K)	Nerve and muscle function, energy metabolism, required for acid–base balance and osmoregulation of the body fluids	Meat, fruit and vegetables	Muscular weakness, retarded development, decreased water intake, inability to maintain water balance, dry skin and alopecia	Greater than normal fluid intake
Sodium (Na)	Muscle and nerve action. Maintenance of osmotic pressure, acid–base and water balance	Common salt, milk, meat, eggs and vegetables	Fatigue, exhaustion, inability to maintain water balance	Greater than normal fluid intake, polydipsia and polyuria can be noted

yoghurt reinforces the gastrointestinal mucosal barrier and helps stimulate gastrointestinal immunity. Questions have been raised on the ability of the bacteria to survive the acidic environment of the stomach. Hence, the use of prebiotics has been stated to be more advantageous than probiotics. Probiotics if administered need to be provided in large enough quantities and potentially on a daily basis. Yeasts have also been included in some probiotic preparations. Their role is to aid in improving the digestibility of fibre and other nutrients. Populations of yeasts do not seem to be maintained within the established gastrointestinal flora, and thus in order to maintain their effect administration on a daily basis is required.

Table 2.7 **The function and source of microminerals, and consequences of deficiencies and excesses**

Micromineral	Function	Source	Deficiency	Toxicity
Copper (Cu)	Formation and activity of red blood cells cofactor in many enzyme systems, and in normal pigmentation (melanin) of skin and hair	Liver, meat, fish	Anaemia, decreased haemoglobin synthesis. Bone disorders can also occur	Can also cause anaemia. Copper toxicosis can occur because of an inherited defect, resulting in hepatitis and cirrhosis
Iodine (I)	Component of the thyroid hormones, which regulate metabolism	Fish, shellfish	Goitre, hypothyroidism. Clinical signs include skin and hair abnormalities, apathy and dullness. Abnormal calcium metabolism and reproductive failure	Acute effects are similar to those of a deficiency. Toxicity can impair thyroid hormone synthesis and produce toxic goitre
Iron (Fe)	An essential component of haemoglobin and myoglobin, present in many coenzymes involved in cellular respiration	Liver, meat, green vegetables	Anaemia with weakness and fatigue	Anorexia and weight loss in dogs
Manganese (Mn)	Required for carbohydrate and lipid metabolism, growth factor in bone development, enzyme activator and component of connective tissue	Liver, kidneys	Defective growth and reproduction. Disturbances in metabolism, especially of lipids	Not reported
Selenium (Se)	An obligatory component of glutathione peroxidase, an antioxidant. Linked with vitamin E, and can replace it to some degree	Meat, offal, cereals	Degeneration of skeletal and cardiac muscles in dogs. In other species, reproductive disorders and oedema	Highly toxic in large doses
Zinc (Zn)	Component of enzyme systems, metabolism of protein and carbohydrates. Essential for maintaining healthy skin and coat	Liver, fish, shellfish	Poor growth, anorexia, testicular atrophy, emaciation and skin lesions. Marginal deficiencies can present as poor skin and coat condition	Relatively non-toxic

The three main mechanisms of action for probiotics are:

■ *Competitive exclusion.* Colonization sites within the gastrointestinal tract and nutrients within the gut are utilized by the probiotics. This thus reduces the availability of resources to the potentially pathogenic bacteria. Chronic gut dysbiosis (when undesirable microorganisms take over in large numbers) can have detrimental effects on the immune system of the digestive system.[3]

Table 2.8 Functions of antioxidants in the body

Antioxidant	Function
Vitamin A	Powerful anticancer and some antiviral properties. Helps maintain the stability of cell membranes
Vitamin E	Protects polyunsaturated fatty acids (PUFA) from peroxidation by free radicals
Vitamin C	Regenerates vitamin E, glutathione and flavenoids
Minerals (selenium, zinc, copper, iron and magnesium)	Selenium is linked with vitamin E. It is a coenzyme of glutathione peroxidase, acting as an antioxidant. The combined effect of vitamin E and selenium is more effective than either alone. High dietary concentrations of copper and iron may be pro-oxidants
Alpha-lipoic acid	Helps to neutralize free radicals, and can be used to treat nerve damage, and help slow the development of ageing and cardiovascular disease
L-Carnitine	When combined with alpha-lipoic acid (in a form known as acetyl-carnitine) the two substances have a synergistic effect, and thus enhance particularly the anti-ageing and energy-producing properties
Glutathione peroxidase	Dependent on selenium and glutathione for its formation. Especially important in reducing the production of inflammatory prostaglandins and leukotrienes

- *Immunomodulation.* A synergistic effect exists between probiotics and the stimulation and functioning of the immune system.
- *Digestive efficiency.* Probiotic microflora has an important role in aiding the breakdown of complex food nutrients.

Prebiotics are specific nutrients that encourage the growth of a beneficial bacterial population (e.g. specific types of fibre). Benefits that the host will experience from this manipulation of the gastrointestinal bacteria include:

- inhibition of potential pathogenic bacteria; this will cause a reduction in endotoxins, carcinogens and substances associated with putrefaction
- stimulation of gastrointestinal immunity
- increased synthesis of vitamins, especially B complex and K
- increased absorption of nutrients
- improved faecal consistency
- increased production of volatile fatty acids (VFA)/short-chain fatty acids (SCFA).

VFA benefit the animal by increasing available nutrients for gastrointestinal bacterial populations, which in turn reduces the quantity of nitrogenous waste materials available to enter the bloodstream and cause azoteamia. This process is sometimes referred to as a nitrogen trap in renal diets. Examples of prebiotics include:

Manno-oligosaccharides (MOS)

MOS are prebiotics that also aid in increasing the populations of certain microflora that benefit the animal. Their unique structure also attracts pathogens and bonds them to the manno-sugars, rather then attaching to the surface of the gut villi.[3]

Glutamine

Glutamine is an amino acid commonly included in critical care nutrition diets, because of its immune-enhancing properties and ability to enhance wound healing. Glutamine is utilized in rapidly dividing cells, like epithelial enterocytes and mucosal immune cells.[3] Glutamine acts as a prebiotic by maintaining the overall health of the gut lining, and therefore ensuring optimal nutrient absorption.[3]

Fructo-oligosaccharides (FOS)

FOS act as a nutrient source for the beneficial bacteria of the gastrointestinal tract (GIT). They also increase gut transit time and draw water into the faeces, increasing bulk and softness.

Energy calculations

To ensure that the patient is receiving sufficient calories, calculations can be performed based on weight. The calculated energy requirement divided by the calorific value of the diet on an 'as-fed basis' will result in the quantity of diet to be fed. Daily weighing of the animal and the use of body condition scores (BCS) will confirm whether the calories provided to the animal are sufficient, adequate or excessive.

Basal energy requirement (BER)
The BER is the amount of energy required by a healthy animal in a thermoneutral environment, whilst awake but not exercising, 12 hours after eating.

Resting energy requirement (RER)
The RER differs from the BER as it includes energy expended for recovery from physical activity and feeding, and the equation used to calculate it depends on the weight of the animal. The RER for dogs and cats can be calculated with these two formulae:

$$RER\ (kcal/day) = 70(BW_{kg})^{0.75} \quad \text{(if bodyweight (BW) is less than 2\,kg)}$$

or

$$RER\ (kcal/day) = 30(BW_{kg}) + 70 \quad \text{(if bodyweight (BW) is between 2–45\,kg).}$$

It has been calculated that RER may be 1.25 × BER, but many texts regard the two as interchangeable values.

In equines the RER is calculated with the formula:[4]

$$RER\ (kcal/day) = 21\ (BW_{kg}) + 975$$

Maintenance energy requirement (MER)
The MER is the energy required for a moderately active adult animal in a thermoneutral environment. This includes energy for obtaining, digesting and absorbing food to maintain an optimal bodyweight. Average values for a dog are 2 × RER, and for cats 1.4 × RER.

Daily energy requirement (DER)
The DER represents the average daily energy requirement for any animal, dependent on lifestage and activity. The DER is calculated from the RER and a lifestage factor.

> Kitten (growth) = 2.5 × RER
> Neutered cat = 1.2 × RER
> Entire cat = 1.4 × RER
> Active cat = 1.6 × RER
> Pregnancy = 1.6–2 × RER
> Lactation = 2–6 × RER (dependent on number of nursing kittens).

Some food manufacturers market different types of foods for neutered male and neutered female cats. There is a metabolic difference between the two sexes, but it is marginal.

> Neutered dog = 1.6 × RER
> Entire dog = 1.8 × RER
> Active/working = 3–8 × RER
> Pregnancy >21 days = 3 × RER
> Lactation = 4–8 × RER (dependent on number of nursing puppies).

All calculations are a rough estimate, and should be adapted to the individual depending on condition scores and weight gain and losses. For illness factors, see Chapter 8.

In calculating energy requirements for equines, many texts use DE requirements for maintenance, as a direct formula:

$$DE\ (MJ/day) = 5.9 + 0.13BW$$

where BW is in kilograms for a normal working horse weighing less than 600 kg. Heavier horses have a lower DE, normally attributed to a lower activity level, and slower rates of acceleration and deceleration during voluntary work.[5] Recalculations are made in order to compensate for these adjustments:[6]

$$DE\ (MJ/day) = 7.61 + 0.1602BW - 0.0000633BW^2$$

Energy metabolism

The route by which energy (adenosine triphosphate; ATP) is obtained from the diet depends on the nutrients absorbed. Calculating the amount of energy from the diet that is ultimately metabolized by the body is dependent on digestibility, the amount of energy lost in urine and faeces, and the energy required in absorbing the nutrients. The gross energy (GE) of the diet is the total heat produced by burning the food in a bomb calorimeter. Subtracting incremental energy losses from the GE will result in the net energy (NE) that can be used by the animal.

References

1. Hotston-Moore P. Fluid therapy for veterinary nurses and technicians. Edinburgh: Butterworth-Heinemann; 2004.
2. Wills JM. Basic principles of nutrition and feeding. In: Kelly N, Wills JM, eds. Manual of companion animal nutrition and feeding. Gloucester: BSAVA Publications; 1996:10–21.
3. Thorne J. To supplement or not to supplement? Part 1. VN Times 2005; (Dec):10–11.
4. Geor RJ. Nutritional support of the sick adult horse. In: Pagan JD, Geor RJ, eds. Advances in equine nutrition II. Kentucky: Kentucky Equine Research; 2001:429–452.
5. Buffington CAT, Holloway C, Abood SK. Manual of veterinary dietetics. St Louis, Missouri: Elsevier Saunders; 2004.
6. Frape DF. Equine nutrition and feeding. 2nd edn. Oxford: Blackwell Science; 1998.

Further and suggested reading

Agar S. Small animal nutrition. Edinburgh: Butterworth-Heinemann; 2001.
National Research Council. Nutrient requirements of domestic animals. Nutrient requirements of horses. 5th edn, revised. Washington, DC: National Academy of Sciences; 1989.

3

Food and feeding

Labelling of diets

In order to correctly identify the diet of choice for an individual, evaluation of the diet needs to be made. This is achieved by analysis of the ingredients. The labelling of pet foods, whether lifestage diets or prescription diets, must contain several pieces of information (Fig. 3.1).

Diets that are fed for a clinical application are required to show further information relating to the particular purpose they are designed for and the species being fed. The type and levels of nutrients and additives, and the characteristics of the diet that have been modified to suit this purpose should be stated. Also stated is the length of time for which the animal should be fed the diet; this is normally 6 months. It is recommended that all patients on clinical diets, on a long-term basis, have a medical examination at least every 6 months. For example, cats on diets designed to prevent feline lower urinary tract disease (FLUTD) should have a urine sample analysed every 6 months, while renal patients should have repeated blood biochemistry and haematology analysis.

Food comparisons

The quality of the food cannot be assessed from the food label, especially the true digestibility of individual nutrients and the overall digestibility of the diet. The bioavailability of nutrients is not disclosed on the label, and this does need to be conveyed to owners when they compare foods. The typical analysis states the percentage of protein, oil (fat), fibre, ash and moisture (when over 14%). In the USA there is a guaranteed analysis, where percentages again are used, but minimum and maximum values of each nutrient are given.

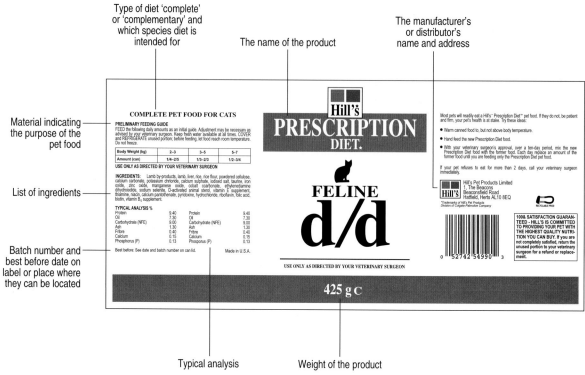

Type of diet 'complete' or 'complementary' and which species diet is intended for

The name of the product

The manufacturer's or distributor's name and address

Material indicating the purpose of the pet food

List of ingredients

Batch number and best before date on label or place where they can be located

Typical analysis

Weight of the product

Figure 3.1 Diagram of a pet food label, demonstrating the legally required information that it must include.

The moisture content of the diet has a direct effect on the remaining ingredients, moist diets being more dilute than dry diets. Thus direct comparison of the typical analysis is inaccurate when moisture contents differ (Box 3.1). Comparisons should only be made when using dry matter basis (DMB) percentages, or when based on energy content (e.g. per 100 kcal).

Proximal analysis of food

The most common method of determining the nutrient content of the diet is through proximal analysis. This method calculates the percentage of water (moisture), protein, fat, ash and crude fibre in the diet. The percentage that is left (i.e., 100% – % moisture – % crude protein – % fat – % crude fibre – % ash) is carbohydrates or nitrogen-free extract (NFE). Crude protein levels are calculated on the basis that protein contains 16±2% nitrogen. The

crude protein therefore equals nitrogen × 6.25, or nitrogen divided by 0.16. Errors can occur when non-protein nitrogen such as urea or ammonia is

> **Box 3.1   Comparison between dry and moist diets when calculated on a dry matter basis (DMB)**
>
> Food A: 75% moisture, 10% protein
> Amount of dry matter (100 – 75) = 25% dry matter
> Protein content = (10/25) × 100 = 40% protein on DBM
>
> Food B: 20% moisture, 10% protein
> Amount of dry matter (100 – 20) = 80% dry matter
> Protein content = (10/80) × 100 = 12.5% protein on DMB
>
> Thus Food A contains over three times as much protein as Food B on a DMB

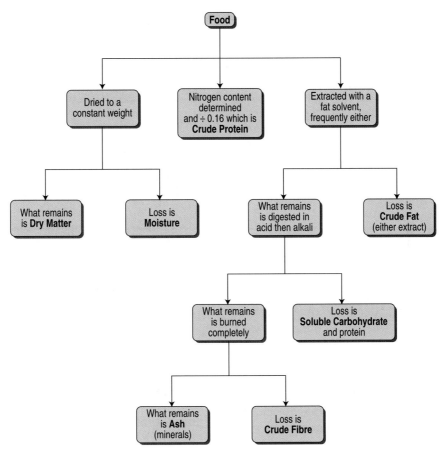

Figure 3.2 Proximate analysis of foods.

used with the product. Figure 3.2 demonstrates proximate analysis of foods.

Types of proprietary diets

Proprietary diets are those that are commercially made, i.e. processed, and fall into two basic categories – complementary or complete.

Complete diets
Complete diets are those that provide a nutritionally balanced and adequate diet when fed as the sole source of food. All of the nutrient components are provided in the correct ratio and do not require addition of any source. In fact adding in large quantities to the diet can make the overall daily intake of food nutritionally unbalanced.

Complementary diets
Complementary diets are those that do not provide a nutritionally balanced diet when fed alone. These diets are designed to be fed in combination with another diet, in order to form a balanced and adequate diet. All treats and snacks are labelled as complementary foods, and thus should only make up a small portion of the daily ration.

Homemade diets

It is still relatively common for cats and dogs to be fed homemade diets. If prepared well, and careful consideration has been made to ensure that they are balanced, homemade diets can serve some purpose in certain cases, e.g. in food trials. Many homemade diets contain excessive quantities of protein and carbohydrates, and are limited in vitamins and minerals, especially calcium. If owners do wish to pursue the use of a homemade diet, examples of a diet should be obtained from the veterinary practice. It is also advisable that the animal has its body condition score (BCS), weight and clinical health examined regularly, to ensure that the diet is balanced and no deficiencies are present. Aiding the owner in designing the diet is important, and there are six simple guidelines to follow when designing a diet.[1] They are:

1. Do the five main food groups appear in the diet?
   - a multivitamin and trace mineral source
   - a source of minerals, especially calcium
   - a fat source
   - a protein source; it is vital in feline diets that an animal-sourced protein is used
   - a carbohydrate source; this also includes fibre. Sources used should be from cooked cereals, grain or potato. (Potatoes are an excellent carbohydrate source when performing food trials, as they are not commonly used in commercial diets.)

2. What is the quality and source of the protein?
   - The protein levels and the protein quality within the diet are two very different elements. A high protein level does not necessarily mean that the animal is receiving all of the essential amino acids it requires. Skeletal muscle protein from different sources contains similar amounts of amino acids, and there is therefore no great advantage of feeding one type of meat over another, unless it is for the purpose of food trials. Novel protein sources used include duck, venison, salmon and egg. Egg is an excellent protein source (BV 100%), and in cases where restricted protein levels are required the inclusion of egg as a protein source in the diet is highly recommended.

3. What is the fat content of the protein source?
   - Cuts of meat vary greatly in their content of fat. Where the fat content is high other fat levels should be reduced in order to compensate for this.

4. What is the carbohydrate to protein ratio within the diet?
   - The carbohydrate to protein ratio should be approximately 1:1 to 2:1 for cat diets and 2:1 to 3:1 in canine diets.[1]

5. Is there a source of vitamin and minerals?
   - A homemade diet will be unbalanced in terms of vitamins and minerals unless these are supplemented. When using homemade diets for food trial cases the use of supplements is not recommended, as this will affect the trial. As the trial is not long term, short-term deficiencies can be tolerated.

6. Is there a source of other essential nutrients?
   - Other essential nutrients such as essential fatty acids (EFA), taurine and other essential amino acids (EAA) do need to be supplemented in the diet. This can be achieved through the addition of oils and other supplements.

Homemade diets should be cooked, as this aids in increasing the overall digestibility of the diet, and reduces the risk of food poisoning. Overcooking will result in a loss of nutrients from the diet, especially vitamins, and the denaturing of proteins. There are a vast number of different homemade diets available on the internet, and they can even be designed for a specific animal and/or clinical disease.

Palatability

Palatability of any diet is essential if the animal is to eat it. Palatability of a food is its degree of acceptability to an animal. There are three essential components to palatability: the pet (species and individual), the environment (owner, home, lifestyle), and the food itself (smell, shape, texture, taste, nutritional composition). The first component, the pet, cannot be altered in order to enhance the palatability of the diet. The second component, the environment, can be changed in some ways. The habits of the owner around feeding time, the designated areas in which the animal is normally fed, the types of bowls used, etc., can all be changed to benefit the animal. Guidance from the veterinary practice should be able to be sourced by the client in order to aid the animal. The third component, the food itself, plays the largest role in palatability, and will be discussed further.

Food aroma and temperature
The temperature of the food does play a huge role in the acceptance of the diet. Cats prefer food that

is near body temperature. This is a direct reflection of their natural diet in the wild. Food which is taken straight from the fridge can be less appealing, as also can foods above 40 °C/104 °F.[2] The aroma of the diet plays a significant role in the animal's willingness to consume the food. Those animals that have a reduced olfactory capacity, such as older animals, sick animals and those on medications that reduce olfactory senses, can have a marked decrease in acceptance of the diet. Cleaning any mucus from the animal's nose will aid acceptance. The use of moist diets can be advantageous; this is due to these diets giving off stronger aromas.

Prehension

The way in which the animal picks up the food in its mouth, and the way in which it eats it have a role in the palatability of the diet. Cats exhibit three different methods of dry food prehension. The most common method is labial prehension. In this method the cat grasps the kibble between the incisors, without the use of the tongue. The second method, supralingual prehension, involves the cat using the dorsal side of the tongue to lap-up the kibbles. The third method, sublingual prehension, occurs when the cat applies the ventral side of the tongue to the kibble, turning the kibble backwards into the mouth. Sublingual prehension is commonly used in brachycephalic breeds, such as Persians. Different kibble shapes have been shown to suit certain types of prehension. For example, almond-shaped kibbles are best suited for cats that use sublingual prehension.

Prehension and kibble shape and size do not seem to be linked in the dog. The kibble shape and size do affect other feeding parameters, including the time taken to eat the diet, and encouraging the dog to chew the kibble rather than swallow it whole.

Taste

Once the animal has smelt the aroma of the food, and picked it up into its mouth, taste is the third stage in food selection and factors that affect the palatability of the diet. Taste perception can be modulated by four factors:

1. *Sex*. It has been found that female dogs are more receptive to sweet tastes than are males.

2. *Age*. Taste sensitivity does decline with age.

3. *State of health*. Some diseases affect taste. These include chronic renal failure, diabetes mellitus, thyroid dysfunction and cranial trauma. Having a blocked nose will also affect the ability to taste.

4. **Drugs**. Tetracycline alters taste perception.

The taste of the diet can be directly influenced by many factors, including the ingredients used, manufacturing practices, storage, pet food preservation systems, packaging, and palatability enhancers.

Texture

The consistency of the diet has large effects on the quantity fed, the palatability (in some cases), the way in which the diet is stored, and packaged, and the methods by which the animal is fed. Cats and dogs prefer meat-based canned products rather than dry expanded diets.[3] This has been attributed to the higher moisture content, and to blood and fluids containing positive palatability factors.[3]

Moist diets

Moist diets contain 70–85% moisture, and are extremely popular. Packaging for moist diets can range from cans to foil trays to pouches. These diets are very palatable, and can lead to overeating and obesity. The moisture content of these diets can prove to be invaluable when trying to increase the water content of the animal's diet, especially in cases of FLUTD.

Semi-moist diets

Semi-moist diets contain around 30% moisture. The diet pieces are formed by the ingredients being cooked, and formed into a paste. The paste is then passed through an extruder and shaped. Acid preservatives are then added in order to inhibit bacterial and fungal growth. Corn syrup is used to coat the pieces to prevent drying out, and removes the availability of the moisture for bacterial and fungal growth. The coating of the syrup makes the pieces very palatable, but totally unsuitable for diabetic patients. Semi-moist diets should not be fed to cats, as they can contain propyl glycol.

Dry diets

Dry diets contain 10–14% moisture, and can be made by a number of different methods. Using a mixture of dry flaked and crushed cereals and vegetables creates meal-type diets. These diets can be beneficial when catering for large numbers of animals, as each individual animal's requirements can be met. Forming the ingredients into a paste and cooking creates an extruded diet. This process involves steam and pressure-cooking. The cooking process can improve the digestibility of the diet, as some nutrients are broken down in the process. The extruded kibbles can then be coated in flavourings and packaged once dried.

Extruded diets tend to be complete and balanced for the lifestage that they are designed for. In some species, extruded and pelleted diets are preferred as they prevent selective feeding, a common problem in meal-type diets, especially in rabbits and small rodents. Extruded diets do increase chewing compared to pelleted diets, thus increasing palatability and increasing positive eating behaviour, no gulping, etc. This eating behaviour also causes an increase in the production of saliva. Extruded diets are ideal for working/performance diets, for any species, as higher fat levels can be utilized.

Post-ingestion effects

The gastrointestinal tract provides many signals related to food ingestion. The distension of the stomach with food stimulates stretch and chemo-receptors. These receptors send vagal signals to the satiety centre. Both positive and negative feedback mechanisms are responsible for regulating food intake. Negative feedback mechanisms such as insulin, serotonin, leptin, neurotensin and glucagons appear to attenuate food intake. Daily administrations of leptin have shown to decrease food consumption, and thus induce weight loss.[4] Positive feedbacks include the activation of the autonomic system during eating. Opioid and dopaminergic neurons are involved in the stimulation of food intake, and aid in the positive reinforcement of food intake.

Feeding behaviours

Finicky feeding behaviour

Fastidious or finicky eating behaviour can make transition to a new therapeutic veterinary diet almost impossible. This commonly occurring eating behaviour is a human-caused problem, resulting from the animal's conditioned expectations for frequent changes in the food variety or flavour. Owners will often describe their pets as finicky eaters if they are seen as intermittent or slow eaters. This can, however, be due to the animal being overfed, or the animal's own autoregulation of food consumption. Assessment of the animal's BCS will confirm whether or not it is consuming sufficient nutrients.

Behavioural modification of the animal to counteract this feeding behaviour is difficult, as it is reliant on the owner. Often the owner is the cause of the initial problem. Removal of the excessive rotation of different brands and flavours to less frequent changes may help resolve the problem. A ritualizing feeding routine will need to be implemented – set meals at a certain time and place using the same brand of food. Some animals which do self-regulate may benefit from ad libitum feeding.

Those animals that have been fed a high-quality, very palatable diet on an ad libitum basis (mainly cats) will expect this unlimited food availability. In order to change its diet, the animal must be made to become dependent on the owner for food. This can be accomplished by offering ad libitum feeding for 2 set hours per day. Once this routine has been established, the old diet should be restricted to 75% of the previous food intake, and the rest of the daily requirement made up with the new diet, placed in a separate bowl next to the old diet.

Food addictions

Food addictions are fairly common, e.g. cats becoming addicted to tinned tuna. Addictions can lead to nutritional deficiencies, or even toxic syndromes. Counter-conditioning behavioural modification is required over a period of time. This modification can occur by adding a distasteful substance to the food that the animal is addicted to, whilst providing a balanced complete diet of the same flavour as the addictive food.

Food aversions

The implications of food aversions are dramatically underestimated in veterinary practice. In some regards it is not advisable to institute dietary changes whilst clinically ill patients are hospitalized. Diets should be introduced in the home environment once the pet is more stable.

Prevention of malnutrition by ensuring adequate nutrient intake is crucial in the management of all medical and surgical cases. The veterinary nurse or technician is crucial in practical measures to improve adequate intake. These practical measures include:

History taking

Talking to the owner can prove to be invaluable. Obtaining information on preferred types and consistency of food, and the animal's eating habits, will contribute towards getting the animal to eat. Cats can be exceptionally fastidious concerning the size, shape and type of bowl or saucer that they eat out of. Wide-rimmed bowls tend to be preferred, so that they have room for their whiskers.

Removal of the clinical problem

Many medical problems, e.g. renal dysfunction can result in changes of appetite and olfaction. Pain associated with dental disease or neoplasia in the mouth will also decrease appetite. Removal of pain or the causal agent will greatly improve the well-being of the patient.

Odorous foods

Warming of the diet to body temperature can prove to be more appetizing to the animal. Increasing the temperature will also increase the odour of the food. Use of highly odorous foods such as pilchards can aid to stimulate eating. None of these measures will work, however, if the animal is unable to smell the food. Any nasal discharges need to be cleaned away before offering the food.

Positive reinforcements

Positive reinforcements such as hand feeding can be used to promote eating. Improving the animal's general well-being, e.g. grooming, can also aid in this process. Trying to encourage eating outside the practice environment can prove to be useful. Taking small quantities of food when exercising the animal outside, or feeding in a room away from all other animals might encourage the animal to eat. Timid animals can benefit from having somewhere to hide away in.

Food aversions can be reinforced by repeatedly offering a diet that the animal keeps refusing.

Force-feeding can be used to aid encouragement to eat, but if the animal becomes distressed this can cause a negative reinforcement to eating that particular food. Any offered food that is not consumed should be removed from the animal's environment after 15 minutes. Littering the animal's cage with a carpet of different foods will not encourage positive eating behaviours.

Feeding methods

The way, in which an animal consumes its diet, does have an impact on many different elements of its life. There are three basic methods of feeding cats and dogs: free choice (ad libitum), time limited or food limited. All have their advantages and disadvantages, and will suit different animals on an individual basis. Significant breed differences have been noted in dogs in their feeding behaviours. Beagles have similar feeding patterns to cats, whereas poodles eat only during the daylight hours. There are, however, always individuals that are exceptions.

Free-choice feeding

This method of feeding does tend to suit those animals that will eat only what is required to meet their energy requirements. Over-consumption can lead to obesity, and during growth in large- and giant-breed dogs can predispose to developmental orthopaedic disorders (DOD). Other disadvantages include food wastage, especially if feeding a moist diet, and competition from other animals in the environment can lead to overeating and consequently undereating in other animals. Advantages include a more constant blood level of nutrients and hormones, and a decrease in coprophagy. Timid animals are more likely to eat, as the longer period of access to food increases their chances of being able to feed when no other animal is present. This method of feeding is advised for animals with or predisposed to FLUTD. This is due to the postprandial alkaline tide; see section on FLUTD in Chapter 18 for more details.

Time-restricted meal feeding

In this method the animal is allowed free access to the food for a set period of time each day. This is usually 10–15 minutes, once or twice daily. This can be a disadvantage in small dogs, puppies and kittens; because of their limited stomach size, insufficient food is consumed to meet their nutritional requirements. Over-consumption can easily occur when using this feeding method, if the animal is greedy. In these cases, reducing the amount of time that the animal has access to the diet, or feeding a diet of a lower energy density, is required. Advantages include aiding in house-training in puppies. A routine of feeding a puppy and then taking it outdoors can enforce house-training by taking advantage of the gastrocolic reflex.

Food-restricted meal feeding

This method requires either calculating the daily energy requirement (DER) of the animal, and thus the quantity of diet that needs to be fed, or following the manufacturer's recommendations on the food packaging. This method of feeding is recommended for animals predisposed to developmental orthopaedic disorders. The calculated DER is then divided by the energy density of the diet in order to obtain the quantity of food that should be fed. The advantage of this diet means that when using a complete balanced diet, the animal is receiving the correct amount of nutrients. The disadvantage is that all animals are individuals, and when initiating this feeding method, reassessment of the quantities fed should be made. Some animals have a higher metabolism or workload and require higher amounts of energy. In these cases a performance diet could be beneficial. On the other hand, some animals may gain weight using this method, and in these cases a light diet could be recommended.

References

1. Tefend M, Berryhill SA. Companion animal clinical nutrition. In: McCurnin DM, Bassert JM, eds. Clinical textbook for veterinary technicians. 6th edn. St Louis, Missouri: Elsevier Saunders; 2006:438–492.
2. Bourgeois H, Elliott D, Marniquet P, et al. The influence of food characteristics on palatability. Focus Special Edition: Dietary preferences of dogs and cats. 2004:23–36.
3. Morris JG, Rogers QR, Fascettis AJ. Nutrition of healthy dogs and cats in various stages of adult life. In: Hand MS, Thatcher CD, Remillard RL, et al., eds. Small animal clinical nutrition. 4th edn. Missouri: Mark Morris Institute; 2000:529–562.
4. LeBel C, Bourdeau A, Lau D, et al. Biological response to peripheral and central administration of recombinant human leptin in dogs. Obes Res 1999; 7(6):577–585.

4
Nutritional assessment

Dogs and cats

There are many recommendations regarding the calculation of an individual's ideal or optimal weight. Recording the animal's weight as a puppy or kitten and throughout the growth phase allows monitoring of the animal's condition. Many practitioners take the animal's weight that was recorded at the time of the first annual vaccination (~1 year old) as the individual's ideal weight. This can be a true reflection, but if the animal was overfed during the growth phase this weight will be an overestimation. Likewise, in larger breeds, maturity and full adult size would not have been reached, and the use of this weight will be an underestimation of ideal bodyweight. Use of breed guidance charts is not advised as there can be huge variations within breeds and it does not take into consideration frame size. When calculating an ideal bodyweight for an individual, the animal must be visibly assessed and palpated. Advising owners on what their animal should weigh if it has never been seen before is not recommended. For example, an owner may phone and ask what is the ideal weight for their terrier, which you have never seen. Use of the body condition score (BCS) index (Fig. 4.1) is the method of choice, but cannot recommend an actual figure for the ideal bodyweight. The BCS can be based on a five-, nine- or ten-point scale. Use of all these different methods, palpating the animal and reassessment after a period of weight gain or loss will provide the best method for calculating an ideal weight. Some breeds do not suit some aspects of the BSC index. For example, whippets and greyhounds in good condition have limited fat cover. Use of a muscle condition score

BCS 1 Emaciated Obvious loss of muscle mass, no body fat or muscle mass. Ribs, spine, pelvic bones easily seen.		
BCS 2 Thin The ribs and pelvic bones are less prominent. Waist and abdomen tuck-up when looking from the side. No palpable fat, but muscle present.		
BCS 3 Moderate (Ideal) Hourglass figure less prominent (waist line), abdominal tuck present. Ribs can be felt but not seen.		
BCS 4 Overweight General fleshy appearance, waistline disappearing. Fat pads starting to form especially at base of tail.		
BCS 5 Obese Sagging abdomen, large fat deposits over the thorax, abdomen and pelvis. Ribs no longer palpable.		

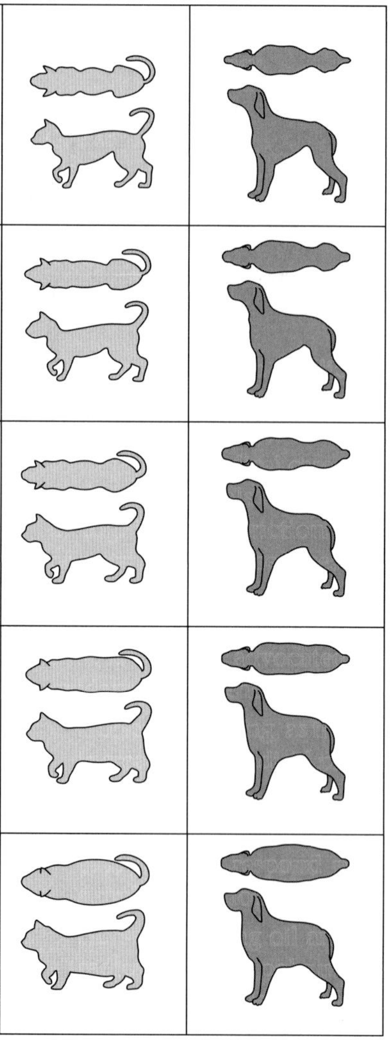

Figure 4.1   Body condition scores.

(MCS; Fig. 4.2) should be utilized alongside the BCS. It is especially important to use the MCS when initiating a weight loss diet, as dramatic losses could be due to a drop in muscle mass and this needs to be prevented.

All of these methods are subjective, but perform the job adequately. Other very sophisticated techniques are currently being used in human patients or in research work (e.g. multiple-frequency bioelectrical impedance, dual-energy radiographic absorptiometry (DEXA), and neutron activation).[1]

'Overcoat syndrome' occurs when a MCS of 1 or 2 is present but the animal is carrying excessive amounts of weight. The large fat deposits mask the muscle wastage that is occurring. This can easily occur in animals that suffer from a dramatic decrease in food consumption, e.g. acute anorexia. Other aspects of physical examination of the patient should be taken into consideration. These aspects include hair coat quality and skin condition, evidence of peripheral oedema or ascites (which may indicate hypoproteinaemia), and clinical signs that indicate certain

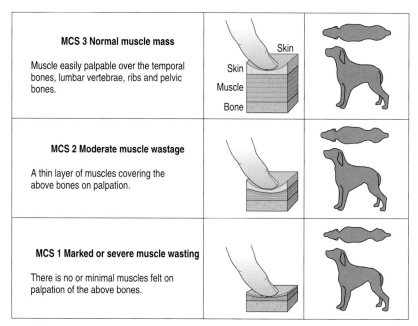

MCS 3 Normal muscle mass Muscle easily palpable over the temporal bones, lumbar vertebrae, ribs and pelvic bones.	Skin Muscle Bone	
MCS 2 Moderate muscle wastage A thin layer of muscles covering the above bones on palpation.		
MCS 1 Marked or severe muscle wasting There is no or minimal muscles felt on palpation of the above bones.		

Figure 4.2   Muscle condition scores.

deficiencies in micronutrients (e.g. neck ventro-flexion or tetany).[1]

Condition scoring of rabbits

Condition scoring for rabbits follows a pattern similar to that of other species (Table 4.1).

Condition scoring of horses

The use of BCS has a vital role in monitoring the health and day-to-day well-being of horses. BCS and weight estimation (WE) are two practical tools that can be utilized when the availability of weighing scales is limited. There are three main BCS in use. The first is the 0–5-point system, as used in dogs, cats and rabbits. The second is the 1–9-point system (mainly used in quarter horses, thoroughbreds and similar breeds), and the third is an adaptation of the second system, but utilized in warmbloods.

The 1–9-point BCS involves each area of the horse being assessed individually and marked accordingly. The six scores are then added together and divided by six in order to give the average BCS for that individual (Table 4.2).[2]

Weight estimations of horses

The estimation of a horse's weight can be performed in number of different methods. The use of a weigh tape can be useful, but the consistency with how the tape is held is important. The use of a weight formula can prove to be very accurate. Again the consistency with which the tape is held is important, and measurements should be in centimetres. The full equations is:

$$Bodyweight\ (kg) = \frac{Girth^2 \times Body\ length\ (cm)}{11\ 877}$$

Body length is measured as the point of shoulder to *tuber ischii* (point of buttock) (Fig. 4.3). In order to

Table 4.1   **BCS for rabbits**

BCS 1 Thin	Loss of muscle, no fat cover, ribs and other bones clearly visible
BCS 2 Ideal	Correct rabbit shape, ribs felt but not seen, no abdominal bulge
BCS 3 Obese	Pronounced fat layers, rounded shape, ribs no longer palpable

Table 4.2 1–9-point BCS assessment sheet for horses

Body condition score	General appearance	Neck	Shoulder	Withers	Thorax	Loin	Tailhead
1	Severely emaciated (no fatty tissue can be palpated)	Individual bone structure visible, exceptionally bony on palpation	Bone structure visibly defined, and sharp on palpation	Razor like, bones easily visible	Skin furrows between ribs, ribs visible	Vertebrae visible	Tailhead and hips very visible
2	Very thin (emaciated)	Individual bones just visible	Bone structure can be outlined	Minimal fat coverage, withers obvious	Prominent ribs. Slightly less depression between ribs	Slight fat covering over vertical and flat spine projections	Tailhead and hipbones obvious to the eye
3	Thin	Some muscle coverage, no raised muscles or fat	Some fat coverage	Thin and accentuated, some fat coverage	Rib outline obvious to the eye. Some subcutaneous fat	Fat build-up halfway on vertical spines, but easily visible	Prominent tailhead. Hipbones appear rounded, but visible
4	Moderately thin	Some fat, not obviously thin	Some fat cover, shoulder not obviously thin	Smooth edges but prominent	Faint outline, visible to the eye	Slight outward ridge along back	Fat can be felt
5	Good	Neck blends smoothly into body with some fat cover	Shoulder blends smoothly into body	Smoothly rounded over top	Ribs cannot be seen, but easily palpable	Back level	Fat around tailhead, beginning to feel spongy
6	Moderately fleshy	Fat can be easily felt	Fat layer can be palpated	Fat can be felt	Fat covering ribs feels spongy	Slight inward crease	Fat around tailhead is soft and palpable
7	Fleshy	Visible deposits or lumps of fat along neck	Build-up of fat behind shoulder	Fat covering withers is firm	The individual ribs can still be palpated	Slight inward crease down back	Fat around tailhead is soft and rounded off
8	Fat	Thickening of the neck is noticeable	Area behind shoulder filled in flush with body	Area along withers filled with fat	Difficult to palpate the ribs	Evident crease down the back	Tailhead very soft and flabby
9	Obese	Bulging fat	Bulging fat	Bulging fat	Patchy fat over ribs	Obvious deep crease down back	Building fat around tailhead

Scores

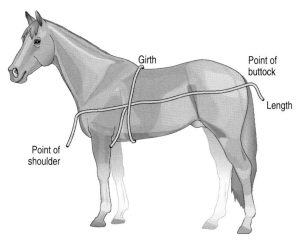

Girth

Point of buttock

Length

Point of shoulder

Figure 4.3 Diagram of points of reference for measurements in order to calculate weight.

gain an accurate estimation of weight the horse must be standing square. The effects of hydration, pregnancy, and weight of intestinal content, etc., are not taken into account when using these methods.[3,4]

Monitoring nutritional interventions

Once an animal has been recommended a specific dietary regimen, it should be reassessed after an appropriate period of time. This depends on the animal, severity of disease (if any present), original nutritional status and the type of nutritional intervention received. Regular weighing of the animal, BCS, MCS and blood haematology and biochemistry parameters can all be utilized in these cases.[1]

References

1. Michel KE. Nutritional assessment. In: Hand MS, Thatcher CD, Remillard RL, et al., eds. Small animal clinical nutrition. 4th edn. Missouri: Mark Morris Institute; 2000:554–555.
2. Harris P, Gee H. Condition scoring and weight estimation: practical tools – 1. Veterinary Review 2005; (Nov):15–18.
3. Harris P, Gee H. Condition scoring and weight estimation: practical tools – 2. Veterinary Review 2005; (Dec):41–43.
4. Carroll CL, Huntingdon PJ. Body condition scoring and weight estimation of horses. Equ Vet J 1998; 20(1):41–45.

section 3

Lifestage Diets

5
Lifestage diets

Lifestage diets of dogs and cats

Gestation and lactation

Recommendations state that, prior to breeding, the bitch or queen needs to be in good condition. This includes nutritional status, that vaccinations are up to date, and any parasiticidal agents are administered (endo- and exoparasiticides). A good body condition score and muscle condition score is required. Bitches and queens that are overweight could possibly present with dystocia during parturition. Obesity, as demonstrated in humans, can also affect fertility. Maintaining bitches during the first 6 weeks of pregnancy on their original adult diet is possible, providing that the diet is of a good quality and is not lacking in any specific nutrients. During the final trimester the bitch will require to be switched to a growth/puppy diet. Large-breed puppy diets are not recommended even for large-breed bitches. These dogs will require a puppy growth diet for dogs under 25 kg. This is due to large-breed puppy diets having a decreased level of energy, which is especially required by the bitch in the last 3 weeks of pregnancy. The bitch's weight should increase to approximately 25% more than that at time of breeding; this does depend, however, on the number in the litter. During this stage more frequent feeding may be required because of a decrease in the quantity of diet consumed at each meal. If the bitch is having difficulties consuming adequate calories, ad libitum feeding should be introduced. Fresh water must be made available at all times.

The feeding of queens during pregnancy differs from that of dogs. Queens increase food intake soon after conception, and this increases with the duration of gestation. During the first third of pregnancy the queen will lay down fat reserves, which will be used towards the end of gestation and during lactation.[1]

Lactation places huge stresses on the nutritional demands of the bitch or queen. The nutritional demands can increase from three to six times that of maintenance. This is dependent on the number in the litter. The growth diet still needs to be fed freely (ad libitum). Large volumes of water will be required and must be available at all times. Peak lactation demands will occur at 3–6 weeks after birth, and further nutritional support of the bitch and queen will be required. Colostrum is vitally important to all mammals; it contains many antibodies from the bitch or queen, aiding in early immunological protection of the puppies or kittens. Queens and bitches sustain a loss of bodyweight during lactation. Ad libitum feeding during pregnancy will allow for the increase in body tissue that will be metabolized during lactation and by fetal energy demands.[2] The weaning bodyweight of the queen or bitch should not be less than the bodyweight at conception.

When nursing, puppies and kittens should be vigorous and active. For the first 3–4 weeks with puppies, and 4 weeks with kittens exclusive feeding from the mother is possible if she is healthy and well nourished. Expected weight gain of kittens should be 10–15 g/day, and puppies 2–4 g/day/kg of anticipated adult weight (or at least 10% gain per day).[2] Puppies and kittens which are not receiving sufficient milk will cry, become restless or extremely inactive and fail to achieve the expected weight gain. It should be remembered that littermates will differ, and gain weight at different rates.

Hand-rearing puppies and kittens

The most obvious alternative to being reared by the mother is by a foster mother. If this is not possible, hand-rearing is the other alternative. Many puppy and kitten formulas are available, and each has its own feeding guidelines. The calorific needs for most nursing-age puppies and kittens are 22–26 kcal per 100 g BW.[2] The quantity of daily feedings is dependent on the formula guidelines, but the formula should be warmed to 37.8°C (100°F) prior to each feeding.

All equipment, bottles, teats, etc., need to be sterilized prior to feeding. In most cases it is more convenient to prepare a 24-hour supply of milk, and divide this into portions required for each meal. Prepared formula must be stored in a refrigerator; any unused prepared formula should be discarded if not used with 48 hours. Chilled prepared formula should not be fed to a puppy or kitten without warming, as colic can be induced. Once fed, the abdomen should appear enlarged but not overdistended.

Tube feeding is another method of feeding orphaned puppies or kittens. If a suckling reflex is present bottle-feeding is the preferred method of choice, due to fewer potential complications. When tube feeding, the formula should be warmed, and administered over a 2-minute period. This will allow sufficient time for slow filling of the stomach.

After feeding, stimulation of the anogenital area is required. This is normally performed with warm moist cotton wool. This provokes the reflexes of micturition and defecation. By 3 weeks of age puppies and kittens are usually able to relieve themselves without simulated stimulation.

A worming regimen of the bitch or queen and of the litter must be implemented, and will have a large effect on the nutritional status and well-being of all. The bitch needs to be wormed prior to breeding and from day 42 of gestation daily until 2 days post-parturition. This is due to transmission of the parasite *Toxocara canis* via both transplacental and transmammary routes. In the queen, worming is only required post-parturition, as transmission of *Toxocara cati* is only transmammary. Studies have shown that a good worming regimen will result in larger healthier puppies and kittens. The offspring will require worming fortnightly from 2 weeks of age, until 12 weeks old.

Weaning

The idea of solids can be introduced to the puppies or kittens from 3 weeks of age. A mixture of the mother's diet mixed with warm water is ideal. At this age the puppies and kittens will show an interest and taste the food, but will not be consuming enough to meet nutritional requirements. Observing the mother eating the diet is important, and will encourage the puppies or kittens to start lapping. When eating their first solid food, kittens do not choose the most palatable food according to innate criteria. They will choose what their mothers eat, even if their food is unusual.[3] From 6–8 weeks of age, complete weaning can start and be achieved. In the majority of cases the bitch or queen will wish to spend less time nursing, and may start to get annoyed or frustrated when puppies/kittens try to suckle.

On weaning, puppies and kittens need to be fed a good-quality complete growth diet. Many breeders have different feeding programmes involving Weetabix, goat's milk, scrambled eggs, mincemeat and calcium supplements. Advising new puppy owners on a correct diet is vital. Questions on what the owners are feeding their pet need to be asked by veterinary practices when the new puppy or kitten is initially presented at the practice. The majority of breeders who use complete growth diets will rehome with the recommendation that the animal remains on the same diet during this transitional period. There is no reason to change the diet unless the animal is not gaining weight adequately, if the diet is not nutritionally balanced or if the animal is grossly overweight.

Feeding puppies and kittens

Puppy growth diets are divided into those designed for pups that will be greater than 25 kg when fully grown, and those that will be less than 25 kg when fully grown. This division is due to growth rates and the age at which maturity is reached. Large breeds should grow at a slower rate over a longer period of time. Diets designed for these breeds are modified with lower energy levels, thus preventing rapid growth rates. Historically these large-breed diets were supplemented with calcium, as it was felt that extra calcium was required to support the skeletal system during the rapid growth rate.[4] Extra calcium is not required, and should be kept in the ratio of 1:1 to 1.5:1 with phosphorus. If the energy content of the diet is correct rapid growth phases are prevented, and the predisposition to developmental orthopaedic disorders (DOD) is reduced. DOD are discussed in more detail in Section 4.

Overfeeding in all puppies and kittens should be avoided, as it can lead to obesity in later life. Slight underfeeding, which does not induce a reduction in full growth potential, will aid in increasing the animal's lifespan. Despite this, high-energy density

is required in growth diets due to the limited capacity of the stomach, and thus the quantity of food able to be consumed in each meal.

Assessment of weight gain needs to be performed on a daily basis for the first few weeks of life. Once weaned and rehomed (normally at 6–8 weeks) puppies and kittens (8–10 weeks) should be weighed at least fortnightly, until 3 months, and then monthly until 6 months old. This conveniently fits in with the required worming regimen. Use of growth charts can be invaluable, and will enable trends in weight gain to be monitored. Too slow a weight gain can reflect insufficient calories being consumed, or that the diet's protein quality is not adequate enough.

Addition of treats to the diet increases greatly during this phase of life, as socialization and training in puppies occurs. Using some of the pup's complete diet kibbles will prevent unbalancing the diet, and can help stop bad feeding habits from being formed. Advice on healthy treat options and other methods of positive reinforcement, i.e. use of toys, social interaction and playing, should be relayed to the owner. The setting up of good feeding habits and behaviour occurs at this age, and puppies and kittens should be introduced to these from an early age.

Docosahexaenoic acid (DHA) has been shown to improve cognitive ability and visual acuity, and has been introduced into commercial puppy and kitten diets. Owing to its benefits, DHA has the potential to speed training, obedience and socialization.

Junior and adolescent diets

Some commercial dog foods offer a junior or adolescent choice of diet. The role of these diets can be beneficial in puppies that require an intermediate diet prior to moving on to an adult maintenance diet. For those brands that do not provide a large-breed puppy diet, utilizing this junior/adolescent diet is necessary to prevent rapid growth rates. When large-breed puppy diets are being fed, changing to a junior or adolescent diet is not required as large-breed puppy diets have a reduced energy content compared with puppy diets.

Adult maintenance

The adult phase is defined from when maturity has been reached until physiological changes occur due to the ageing process. The age at which the adult phase starts depends mainly on breed variations. Smaller breeds can reach full maturity from 6 months, larger and giant breeds from 1 year to 18 months. Each animal should have the diet altered to meet its individual needs. The quantity of diet fed will depend on the quality of the diet, amount of exercise the animal receives, neutering status and metabolism. Those breeds that are predisposed to weight gain should have their weight, BCS and MCS monitored throughout this life phase. Changes of metabolism post-neutering should be noted to owners, and use of 'light' diets or diets specifically aimed at neutered animals should be advocated. These diets are designed to prevent weight gain, not aid in weight loss.

Neutered adult diets

Many diets have now been introduced to the market specifically designed for neutered cats. As previously discussed, after neutering the animal's metabolism decreases. In entire cats energy expenditure in both female and male animals is 57 ± 2 kcal/kg. Once neutered, this value decreases to 50 ± 3 kcal/kg in males,

and 51 ± 2 kcal/kg in females. There are, however, marked differences in other factors as demonstrated in Table 5.1. Changes in insulin resistance can suggest predisposition of neutered cats to diabetes mellitus.

Performance and working diets

Animals that have a high energy expenditure will benefit from a diet with a higher energy density. Because of the stomach's limited capacity, insufficient quantities of the diet may be consumed. The digestive system's capacity and digestive and absorption abilities can be a limiting factor. Care should be taken during periods of reduced activity levels, as excessive calories will result in quick weight gain. High-energy-dense diets are also beneficial for those animals that have a high metabolism and thus find weight gain difficult. When changing any animal to a high-energy-dense diet, a longer than normal transitional period may be required. This is due to the dog's digestive mechanisms having to adjust to this diet. The extra energy required in these diets is supplied in the form of increased fat content, while there is a decrease in fibre content. This increase in energy content is due to the increased calories per

Table 5.1 Difference between male and female cats, and the consequences of neutering[6]

Parameter	Male	Female	Consequence of neutering
Body fat (as % of total bodyweight)	23.8 ± 1	30.1 ± 1.7	Increase M: 32.9 ± 1.7 F: 35.5 ± 1.8
Energy expenditure (kcal/kg)	57 ± 2	57 ± 2	Decrease M: 50 ± 3 F: 51 ± 2
Non-esterified fatty acids		Higher in the female	Greater differences between males and females
Caloric requirements			Requirements reduced in both sexes
Serum leptin	Regulation of leptin secretion by testosterone	No demonstrated oestrogenic control in cats	M: Increase in the male F: Less noticeable change
Glucose intolerance		Absent	Unchanged in both sexes
Insulin	More marked		Continuance of high insulin resistance in the male, whereas in the female appearance of insulin resistance

unit of weight the fat contains. The reduction of fibre is required, as this will increase the digestibility of the diet, and reduce the effect that fibre has on reducing adsorption of other nutrients.

Breed-specific diets

Many commercial diets are now aimed at specific breed types or size. Small-breed diets tend to have a higher energy density compared to those aimed at medium and large breeds. This is due to the small capacity of the stomach, and an increase in metabolism. Care should be taken for those small-breed dogs that put on weight easily, and in some cases small-breed diets might not be the diet of choice. Kibble size is also altered depending on the size and breed of dog for which it is designed. In feline diets, kibble shape has also been shown to affect the way in which certain breeds consume their diet. Persian cats benefit from an almond-shaped kibble, because of the shape of their skull.

Diets aimed at reducing the risk of certain breeds' disposition to certain disorders/diseases have been introduced onto the nutritional market. Diets aimed specifically at Bedlington terriers are now commonplace, and have reduced copper levels.

Senior diets

The senior or geriatric phase of life starts at varying ages related to breed size and species. Toy and small-breed dogs enter the senior stage of life at approximately 8 years, medium breeds at 7–8 years, with large and giant breeds entering a senior lifestage at 5 years. Cats are deemed as senior from 8 years. Other factors such as nutritional status, environment, genetic make-up and clinical health will affect these ages and the longevity of the dog or cat. Changes that occur with age include greying of the muzzle and slowing down in activity levels, but less obvious changes include alteration in the physiology of the digestive tract, immune system, kidneys and other organs. Generally, the capacity to absorb and utilize nutrients is not decreased in older animals, but the body does become less able to tolerate excesses and borderline deficiencies, and the ability to respond to dietary changes may also be decreased.[5] 'Geriatric' screening should be considered in all animals upon reaching a senior age. A critical part of this screening should include evaluation of nutrition.

Table 5.2 Average maintenance energy requirements for dogs at different lifestages

Age (years)	Kcal ME/kg BW$^{0.75}$	KJ ME/kg BW$^{0.75}$
1–2	132	550
3–7	115	480
>7	100	415

ME, metabolizable energy; BW, bodyweight.

Nutritional changes in the diet of the cat or dog are aimed at supporting the physiological changes that occur within this lifestage. Energy requirements for senior dogs are reduced (Table 5.2), due to a decrease in activity levels and expenditure. Some active senior animals may require an energy density higher than that provided by senior diets, and a compromise between senior and adult maintenance is required.

In cats, however, the maintenance energy requirements do not decrease as they get older.[6] This could be due to cats remaining relatively inactive throughout their adult life. It is difficult to differentiate between an older and younger cat simply by looking at activity levels, as cats spend a large portion of their day sleeping. The proportion of obese cats tends to increase until the age of 7. After this it decreases, especially after the age of 10 years.[7]

A reduction in renal function should be considered in all senior animals; a reduction in protein quantities within the diet could be beneficial if renal damage has occurred. The quality of the protein should be increased as skeletal muscle mass reduces, which also reduces any protein or amino acid reserves if required. Some lifestage diets do not have a decrease in protein levels, as some views are that restricted protein levels are not required until there is direct evidence of renal impairment. In fact protein requirements sufficient to support protein turnover actually increase in older dogs and cats. Protein restriction in feline senior diets should be avoided. Cats are especially sensitive to decreases in protein levels within the diet. This is due to their inability to downgrade protein metabolism pathways. Reduced protein digestibility is also experienced in geriatric cats. In healthy adult cats protein digestibility is typically 85–90%. In geriatric cats this digestibility can be reduced to less than 77%.[8]

Diets that have a severely restricted protein level or proteins of a low quality/biological value can predispose cats over 12 years to negative nitrogen balance, and loss of lean body mass.[8]

The restriction of phosphorus in the diet plays a significant role in the prevention of renal impairment. A decrease in kidney function can also lead to an increased loss of the water-soluble vitamins, due to the kidney's decreased ability to concentrate the urine. This can also lead to a reduction in hydration levels of the animal. Senior animals have a reduced sensitivity to thirst, and thus there is a greater risk of dehydration in these animals.[9]

Most senior diets are formulated to have softer kibbles in order to accommodate any dental problems, reduction in number of teeth, and a drop in musculature of the jaw. Moving to a moist diet can benefit the animal if it is having difficulties in mastication. A moist diet will also aid hydration levels.

The use of antioxidants for senior animals has been advocated because free radical production can increase with age, as the diseases associated with ageing (cardiovascular, arthritis) will further increase production of free radicals. Older cats and dogs should be evaluated for vitamin and mineral deficiencies. Owing to oxidative damage, demand of the antioxidant vitamins is greater. Geriatric animals, especially cats, have a reduced ability to digest fats. Because of the association of fat digestibility with the digestibility of other essential nutrients (fat-soluble vitamins), deficiencies can occur.[3]

As the animal ages, smell is the first sense to decline. As the animal's sense of smell deteriorates the animal may eat less. The aroma of the diet is particularly important in diets aimed at senior animals in order to encourage consumption.

Carnivore vs omnivore

Both cats and dogs are formally classed as carnivores. The metabolism and nutritional needs of the dog do approach that of the omnivore classification. Dogs have the ability to synthesize taurine, arachidonic acid and vitamin A from the metabolic precursors cysteine, linoleic acid and beta-carotene respectively. Cats, however, are obligate carnivores and require these specific nutrients in a preformed state from a meat-based diet.

Rabbit lifestage diets

Lifestage diets are now commonly available on the commercial market. All of these diets are designed to be complementary, and fed alongside grass and hay. Rabbits have a low requirement for fat in their diets, 1–2% is ideal. Any fat within a diet needs to be of vegetable origin. Animal fats contain cholesterol that can cause the rabbit to develop atherosclerosis-like symptoms.[10] A recommended protein level for an adult maintenance diet is 12–14%. Animals that require high energy levels due to physical, environmental and psychological stressors may require a protein level of 16–22%. A fat level of 1% and fibre content of 20% is often quoted. Changes in the way in which rabbits are now kept should be remembered. House rabbits are now commonplace, as also is neutering. Neutering has an effect on metabolism that is similar to its effect in cats and dogs. Rabbit caretakers should be made aware of this, as obesity can occur, and prevention is better than cure.

There are many different opinions surrounding which vegetables are suitable for rabbits. The majority of sources agree carrots, carrot tops, broccoli and parsley to be safe. Carrots are considered safe, but should only be fed in small amounts owing to the high sugar content. Other vegetables that have also been used include dandelions, turnip greens, spinach, kale and Romaine lettuce. Beans, potatoes and some lettuces are potentially problematic. Recommended guidelines for the amount of vegetables given daily are to feed at least three types of greens (along with carrot, if wished). It is important to feed more than one type of vegetable in order to prevent nutrient imbalances. The use of a complementary pelleted diet can aid in reducing imbalances. Some vegetables contain high levels of oxalates (kale, mustard greens and spinach). Instead of removing them from the diet altogether, as there are benefits, their use should be limited to one to three meals per week. If you are advising a rabbit caretaker (rabbit owners prefer caretaker) on increasing the vegetable content of the rabbit's diet, it is exceptionally important to stress that changes should be made slowly. Also, that vegetables should be washed thoroughly before offering them to the rabbit. The proportions of diet constituents for the rabbit are usually shown in the form of a feeding pyramid, and make a good visual aid for rabbit caretakers.

Rabbits should not be fed high-sugar treats, i.e. chocolate drops. Treats for rabbits do exist; examples include small amounts of dried foods such as raisins. These must be fed in very small quantities, but in reality the rabbit does not need them in its diet. Chocolate is poisonous to rabbits and should not be fed; yoghurt drops have very high sugar content. Other foods that should be avoided include pasta, bread, biscuits, crackers and breakfast cereals.

Young rabbits

Alfalfa can be fed to young bunnies under the age of 6 months since it provides extra calcium necessary for growing bones. It is important to offer timothy hay as well, so when it comes time to wean them to strictly grass hay they will know the taste and be less likely to resist change. Pelleted lifestage diets tend to contain higher levels of alfalfa, and thus an increase in calcium levels. Up to the stage of sexual maturity, which tends to be around 6 months of age, a diet containing 16–18% protein, 3% fat and 16–18% fibre is required in order to allow for growth and development.

Young rabbits are only fed once daily by their mother, as the mother's milk is exceptionally high in fat. Feeding in this manner will also reduce the risk of predators locating the nest. The young rabbits will start to be interested in solids at roughly 2 weeks of age, and will consume what the doe is eating. The act of caecotrophy usually starts at around 3 weeks of age. A healthy mixture of greens, hay and pellets is recommended as it will encourage the young rabbits to have a varied diet. Complete weaning occurs at 5–6 weeks of age; when the young are rehomed it is recommended that they are fed exactly the same diet as when with the doe. Any dietary changes must occur very slowly; the stress of separation can also act as a factor in digestive upset. Once the young rabbit has completely settled in, then any required dietary changes should be made.

Senior rabbits

At present there are no lifestage diets designed for older rabbits. The diet of these rabbits should reflect any clinical problems usually associated with older age. Weight loss is commonly encountered, but the cause of the weight problem is rarely defined. In some cases the use of alfalfa can be helpful as it has a higher energy density and is slightly more enticing to eat than grass hay. Those animals with dental problems would benefit from vegetables cut slightly smaller, or moistened pellets, in order to aid an adequate nutrient intake. In cases where the animal appears in pain, the use of analgesia should be highly recommended. In many cases, stiffness/lameness is ignored by the owner because of the animal's age.

Equine lifestage diets

The principal function of feed is to provide the nutrient requirements of the horse and its symbiotic gastrointestinal (GI) microorganisms.[11] Nutrition for each lifestage will be discussed, but it should be remembered that requirements differ greatly with bodyweight, digestive efficiency, health status and different physiological demands, i.e. growth, lactation, physical activity, and work load (rider weight and ability, terrain and intensity of activity).[11] The total amount of feed should be adjusted according to all these factors and the nutritional status of the animal (Table 5.3).[12]

Foals

The large intestine of the foal is relatively small, and is therefore dependent on an energy source from digestible starches and simple sugars. In order to aid in stimulation of development of the large intestine, high-quality leafy hay can be fed in small but increasing quantities to act as the required stimulant.[11] Because of this, a daily dietary source of vitamin B_{12} should be provided, until the hindgut bacterial populations are sufficient to satisfy nutrient requirements. It is also recommended that vitamins A, D_3 and E should be supplemented. Foals that have a good growth rate with mares on pasture (Fig. 5.1), do not require any additional dry/concentrate feed. This is until 2–3 months prior to weaning, when creep feeding can be introduced. Protein requirements in foals are high, with the mare's milk being high in levels of lysine.

Weanlings

Foals are under a large amount of stress at the time of weaning, due to a change in their diet, the loss

Table 5.3 **Minimum daily nutrient requirements of horses**[12]

	Digestible energy (MJ)	Crude protein (g)	Lysine (g)	Calcium (g)	Phosphorus (g)	Magnesium (g)	Potassium (g)
Maintenance (adult)	69	656	23	21	14	7.5	25.0
Stallions (breeding)	86	820	29	26	18	9.4	31.2
Pregnant mares:							
9 months	76	801	28	36	26	8.7	29.1
10 months	77	815	29	36	27	8.9	29.7
11 months	82	866	30	38	28	9.4	31.5
Lactating mares:							
Foaling to 3 months	118	1427	50	57	36	10.9	46.0
3 months to weaning	102	1048	37	38	22	8.6	33.0
Working:							
Light	86	820	29	29	18	9.4	31.2
Moderate	103	880	31	32	21	11.3	37.4
Intense	137	1050	37	40	29	15.1	49.9
Foal growing at 1.0 kg/day:							
4 months	60	730	30	37	19	4.0	11.3
6 months	71	864	36	40	20	4.6	13.3
Yearling growing at 0.6–0.8 kg/day	87	956	40	40	20	5.7	18.2
24 months old:							
Not in training	79	820	32	28	14	7.0	23.1
In training	110	1050	41	35	19	9.8	32.2

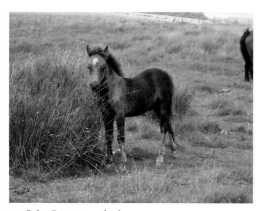

Figure 5.1 Dartmoor foal.

of companionship with their mother, and the possibility of moving to a new location. This stress can manifest as injury, weight loss and illness. The use of creep feeding has been shown to reduce stress on foals at weaning. Creep feeding is given shortly prior to the weaning period, and aids in accustoming the foal's digestive tract to non-milk feeds. Healthy foals will start to nibble at hay and concentrates at 10–20 days of age.[11] In situations where the milk supply or amount of grass is inadequate, the utilization of creep feeds can be initiated, and normal growth in the foal can be achieved. Prior to weaning the dam should be removed from high-quality pasture, and any supplementation of the diet stopped. This will limit milk secretion. After weaning the udder should not be milked out. The use of creep feeding should be advocated, not only for reducing the stress associated with dietary changes, but also for reducing the potential for post-weaning developmental orthopaedic disorders. A specific diet for weanlings is difficult to suggest, because of body size and nutrient requirement differences, differences in pasture and hay quality and environmental conditions. The most important aspect of the diet is that it should contain 1.5–2.5 times more calcium than phosphorus.[12] The use of milk pellets as a creep feed before weaning is contraindicated as it defeats the prime objective.[13] Supplementary creep feed should be restricted to 0.5–0.75 kg/100 kg BW.[13] Overfeeding of foals is easily done, and can lead to DOD. A restriction of concentrates will give a measure of control over the incidence of these growth-associated ailments. Studies conducted into weaning foals have found that those with access to a pasture supplement based on fat and fibre were more relaxed than foals of a similar age fed on a more traditional supplement rich in starch and sugars.

The performance horse

Diet has the potential to delay or reduce the onset of muscle fatigue by protecting against oxidative stress and dehydration, alongside electrolyte imbalances. Energy is the nutrient that is most affected by exercise, and depending on the nature and intensity of work will alter the horse's daily energy requirements. Starch is a versatile energy source for the performance horse, and can be used in a number of different ways; either oxidized directly to produce ATP or used to make muscle glycogen, liver glycogen or body fat.[14] Starch is the dietary energy source of choice for glycogen synthesis, but there is a limit to the quantity of starch that should be present in the diet. High dietary starch levels can overwhelm the functioning of the small intestine. Insufficient absorption can occur, allowing a substantial quantity of starch to pass through into the large intestine. This can result in rapid fermentation, and lactic acid production, which in turn will cause a decrease in the hindgut pH.

The requirement of fibre in the diet should not be overlooked. Due to the highly developed hindgut, suitable fibre sources are required in order to sustain the microorganisms present. Hay should be fed at a rate of intake equal to at least 1% of bodyweight per day.[14]

Fat supplies higher levels of calories in a concentrated form than carbohydrates and proteins. Addition of fats to the diet needs to occur slowly as the horse's GI system adapts to the dietary changes. Horses will digest over 90% of vegetable oils in a diet, even when fed at levels over 500–600 ml per day.[14] Quantities of oil to be included in the diet are highly dependent on the animal's energy expenditure. In horses, where beneficial effects on hair coat are required, 70–80 ml of oil per day is recommended. This will only provide 2.5% of a lightly exercised horse's digestible energy (DE) requirement.[14] Horses in heavy training will require levels of ~ 450 ml of vegetable oil per day.[14] This relates to roughly 10% of its total daily DE intake, and roughly 20% of the DE supplied by the concentrates. Very high levels of fat in the diet (>500 g/ day) have been shown to compromise muscle and liver glycogen storage.

Protein in excess of the animal's daily requirements can be used as an energy source. Excessive protein levels should be avoided, however, for three specific reasons:

- Water requirements increase with increased protein intake.

- An increase in blood urea nitrogen (BUN) levels will result in an increase in urea excretion into the gut. This may increase the risk of intestinal disturbances such as enterotoxaemia.

- Blood ammonia increases, causing a number of complications such as nerve irritability and disturbances in carbohydrate metabolism.[14]

Supplemental electrolytes are an important constituent of the performance horse's diet. Electrolytes can aid in the prevention of 'tying-up', help recovery from hard work, and help to begin the necessary rebuilding phase that occurs after exertion.[15] Table 5.4 demonstrates the daily requirements of some electrolytes for horses working at different intensities.

The timing and composition of pre-exercise meals will affect metabolism during exercise.[16] In thoroughbred racehorses, reducing the hay intake to 1% BW for a 3-day period prior to racing will effectively reduce bodyweight, without causing

Table 5.4 **Daily requirements for electrolytes of horses exercising at different work intensities (g/day)**[15]

	Work intensity			
Electrolyte	*Rest*	*Light*	*Moderate*	*Heavy*
Sodium	10	20	50	125
Chloride	10	25	70	175
Potassium	25	30	44	75
Magnesium	10	11	14	15–19

any digestive disturbances. Feeding a glycaemic meal before racing may also increase glycogen utilization and increase power output during the race.[16] With endurance horses, bodyweight is not of concern, and therefore forage intake should be high before an event. Fat oxidation is the main source of energy in these animals, and therefore feeding grain 1–4 hours prior to a ride should be avoided, as elevated insulin levels will suppress the oxidation of fats. However, immediately before exercise, grain can be fed as it will not disrupt fat utilization, since exercise-induced elevation in epinephrine (adrenaline) depresses the release of insulin.[16] Care must be given in not predisposing to colic, though no direct evidence has been found of the influence of a full stomach and exercise on the risk of colic.[17] The horse's stomach is very well attached to the abdominal wall, and is capable of little movement, so the risk of colic associated with movement of a full stomach is very small.[17] A full stomach will slow down a racehorse and have some effect on respiratory function, as it will affect ability of the lungs to fill.[17]

The feeding of three-day event horses will depend on the activity that is about to be performed, or just being recovered from. As with endurance horses, the withholding of grain before the speed and endurance day is beneficial, as it will stimulate fat utilization. A reduction in muscle glycogen levels may affect the horse's ability in the final day events (show jumping). Feeding the horse a high-glycaemic meal or administering glucose after completion of day 2, will aid in a quicker restoration of muscle glycogen stores.[16]

Stud horses

Gestation and parturition

During gestation, maintenance energy levels are adequate up until the last 90 days when approximately 60–65% of the fetal tissue develops. Energy requirements are estimated to be 1.5 times that of maintenance. As the fetus increases in size, there is a proportionate decrease in available space for the abdominal contents. The mare's capacity for bulky feed declines during this period in which nutrient requirements increase.[13] These extra nutrients can be supplied by improving the quality of grazing or the quality of forage if fed on hay and concentrates. Nutrient requirements during this phase will also greatly depend on whether the mare has a foal at foot. The increase in month 11 of gestation is also to sustain udder development. Crude protein requirements for mares in the last 90 days of gestation are ~72 g/kg, based on diets with 90% dry matter (DM).[13]

Calcium and phosphorus levels are of importance during gestation. There is an increase in the demand for calcium, especially peri-parturition during mammary calcium secretion.[13] Recommended levels of calcium and phosphorus through the last 90 days of gestation are respectively 5.5 g/kg and 3.0 g/kg of feed based on 90% DM.[13] These mineral concentrations can be achieved by pasture alone, if it is of a good quality. In the UK, neither grasses nor legume hays provide sufficient quantities. A supplement of dicalcium phosphate, steamed bone meal or wheat bran is required.

Body condition score (BCS) and weight of the mare during gestation are important. Those that are overweight or obese are potentially at a higher risk of complications during parturition. This can include birth difficulties due to less activity and thus poorer muscle tone and delayed expulsion of the placenta. An ideal BCS and weight should be achieved prior to breeding, and maintained throughout gestation. Corrections to BCS and weight should not be obtained during gestation, as restrictions on fetal growth can occur.

Twenty-four hours prior to the birth of the foal, good-quality hay alongside a low-energy cereal mixture including bran, or commercial pony nuts, should be fed, in a light meal.[13] Warm water should be available to the mare at all times. The first meal after parturition should be a bran mash; the second meal can have the inclusion of good-quality stud nuts or cereal–protein mixture. Protein content of these feeds should be around 16–17%, with around 3% oil and 8% crude fibre.[13] Restrictions should be made on the quantity of concentrates fed to mares during the first 10 days, in order to avoid excessive milk secretions, and digestive disturbance in the foal.

Lactation

Lactation places large demands on the dam. The protein content of the milk is at its highest level immediately post-parturition, and declines gradually throughout lactation. Milk production, however, increases throughout as the foal demands more. High-quality proteins are therefore required for the dam during the stage of lactation. Milk yields will be influenced by water availability, intake of nutrients and energy, and the horse's own innate ability. The mare's dietary consumption of proteins will directly influence the quality of the proteins present in the milk. Mares that have a decreased protein and fat intake will have increases in protein and fat levels within the milk, but alongside an overall decrease in yield.

The stallion

Energy requirements of the stallion will differ during the calendar year, depending on breeding seasons. The BCS of the stallion is important to be maintained throughout the year, whether breeding or not. During breeding seasons the energy requirement of the stallion will increase, as more is expended. This is mainly due to nervous energy expended, and that utilized when pacing his stall or run. Dietary changes will be required, but levels required will be dependent on the individual horse. There has been no direct evidence that specific dietary supplements will enhance the fertility of stallions. A good-quality balanced diet, with the stallion at a good BCS, is the most efficient way to maintain the fertility of the stallion.[13]

The older horse

The event of old age in horses is viewed differently than in other companion animals. It has been stated that just because a horse is over 16 years old does not mean that it is geriatric.[18] Horses with good BCS that are active and healthy should not have their dietary routine changed. Rations for the older horse should provide at least:

- 12% protein
- restricted calcium (<1.0%)
- marginally increased phosphorus (0.3–0.5%); the calcium to phosphorus ratio should be greater than 1:1
- crude fibre content above 7%.

In cases where dentition is becoming a problem, alterations to the diet can occur. Gruels of soaked hay cubes or beet pulp can be utilized, alongside pellets, micronized or extruded feeds specifically designed for the older animal. Plenty of water must be made available so that constipation/impaction problems can be reduced.[18]

Horses that do not have a reduced renal function can benefit from a diet that is similar to those recommended for weanlings, compared to those for adult maintenance. Some horses will not require older-horse rations, because of their performance levels, and this should therefore be taken into consideration. When older horses do retire, the energy levels of the diet need to be altered in order to compensate for this.

References

1. Debraekeleer J. Nutrition of the aging dog: How can we improve quality of life? Veterinary Times 2005; (31 Jan):10–12.

2. Morris JG, Rogers QR, Fascetti AJ. Nutrition of healthy dogs and cats in various stages of adult life. In: Hand MS, Thatcher CD, Remillard RL,

et al., eds. Small animal clinical nutrition. 4th edn. Missouri: Mark Morris Institute; 2000:555–560.

3. Wyrwicka W. Imitation of mother's inappropriate food preference in weanling kittens. Pavlov J Bio Sci 1978; 13(2):55–72.

4. Harper EJ. Changing perspectives on aging and energy requirements: aging and energy intake in humans, dogs and cats. J Nutr 1998; 128:2623–2626.

5. Furniss G. Puppy and kitten nutrition. VN Times 2006; (June):26–28.

6. Laflamme DP. Nutrition for ageing cats and dogs, and the importance of body condition. Vet Clin Small Anim 2005; 35(3):713–742.

7. Dethioux F, Marniquet P, Petit P, et al. How can we prevent the metabolic consequences of neutering? Focus Special Edition: Preventative nutrition for major health risks in cats. 2005:9–18.

8. Kelly M, Jean-Phillippe C, Cupp C. Advances in nutritional care of the older cat. VN Times 2006; (June):8–9.

9. Hoskins JD. Neonatal and pediatric nutrition. In: Ettinger SJ, Feldman EC, eds. Textbook of veterinary internal medicine. Volume 1. 6th edn. St Louis, Missouri: Elsevier Saunders; 2005:561–562.

10. TeSelle E, McBee C. Natural nutrition Part II: Pellets and veggies. House Rabbit Society; 2006. Online. Available: http://www.rabbit.org

11. Harris PA, Frape DL, Jeffcott LB, et al. Equine nutrition and metabolic disease. In: Higgins AJ, Wright IM, eds. The equine manual. London: Saunders; 1995:123–186.

15. National Research Council. Nutrient requirements of domestic animals. Nutrient requirements of horses. 5th edn, revised. Washington, DC: National Academy of Sciences; 1989.

16. Frape DF. Equine nutrition and feeding. 2nd edn. Oxford: Blackwell Science; 1998.

17. Pagan JD. Energy and the performance horse. Proceedings of the BEVA Specialist Days on Behaviour and Nutrition; September 1999:60–62.

18. Pagan JD. Vitamins, trace elements and electrolytes for the performance horse. Proceedings of the BEVA Specialist Days on Behaviour and Nutrition; September 1999:63–66.

19. Pagan JD. Time of feeding critical for performance. Dodson and Horrell Ltd 3rd International Conference on Feeding Horses. Scientific Session; 2000:58–65.

20. Proudman C. Feeding to avoid colic. Dodson and Horrell Ltd 5th International Conference on Feeding Horses. Applied Session; 2005:51–56.

21. Ralston SL. The older horse: diet and health care. Dodson and Horrell Ltd 4th International Conference on Feeding Horses. Applied Session; 2002:37–42.

Suggested reading and information sources

Agar S. Small animal nutrition. Edinburgh: Butterworth-Heinemann; 2001.

Frape D. Equine nutrition and feeding. 2nd edn. Oxford: Blackwell Science; 1998.

House Rabbit Society website. www.rabbit.org

section 4

Clinical Nutrition

6
Cancer

Nutrition can play an important role in the 'prevention' and treatment of cancers. This does, however, vary with the type of tumour and stage of progression. The potential risk reduction of cancer when following dietary recommendations has not been well documented in veterinary medicine. In human studies 'eating right', staying active and maintaining a healthy weight can reduce the risk of cancer by 30–40%.[1] It has been speculated that this reduction may be even more achievable in pets as their dietary intake can be more controlled. Correct feeding of the cancer patient can enhance quality and length of life. This is due to nutritional support reducing or preventing toxicoses associated with cancer therapy and ameliorating cancer-induced metabolic alterations. Anorexia is a common clinical symptom in cancer patients, which can lead to weight loss and cachexia in conjunction with the metabolic alterations. Use of body condition scores can be an excellent monitoring tool to assess the overall nutritional effect of cancer and treatments. Cancer affects the nutritional status of the animal in three ways:

1. Therapy (e.g. chemotherapy-induced anorexia, nausea or vomiting). Human chemotherapy patients have reported changes in taste and smell. These side effects experienced during therapy make it difficult for some patients to consume optimal quantity of calories and nutrients.

2. Alterations of the metabolic pathways.

3. Tumours can also have a primary effect such as compression or infiltration of the alimentary canal.

Cancer cachexia

Cachexia is defined as a profound and marked state of general ill health and malnutrition. It is a complex paraneoplastic syndrome that includes progressive weight loss that occurs despite adequate nutritional intake.[1] Loss of both fat and muscle can occur with the depletion of muscle mass often exceeding that of viscera in cancer patients. Cachexia is not common in veterinary cancer patients, but weight loss usually occurs early in the course of the disease. Cachexia can cause a decreased quality of life, a decreased response to therapies and shortened survival time, when compared to those with similar diseases without cachexia. Cancer cachexia may be partly due to a negative energy balance (Fig. 6.1). It is therefore important for the owner to have the animal weighed and body condition scored on a regular basis.

The aim of nutritional management is to:

- provide an energy source for the patient, that the tumour cannot readily utilize
- meet the increased nutritional requirements of proteins
- limit lactate production by the tumour

- improve immune function, remission and survival times
- aid in limiting tumour growth.

Clinical nutrition

Carbohydrates

The metabolism of carbohydrates is greatly altered in dogs with cancer. The alteration in metabolism is due to tumours metabolizing glucose via anaerobic glycolysis to lactic acid. A net energy gain by the tumour, and net loss by the host results as the host expends energy converting the lactate back to glucose by the Cori cycle. The alterations in metabolism are suspected, but not yet proven in cats. Hyperlactataemia can result and this should be taken into consideration if intravenous fluid therapy is required. Hartmann's (lactated Ringer's) solution can exacerbate any hyperlactataemia and energy demands.

Carbohydrates can be poorly utilized due to peripheral insulin resistance; excess dietary soluble carbohydrates need to be avoided. Nitrogen-free extract (NFE) needs to be ≤25% of dry

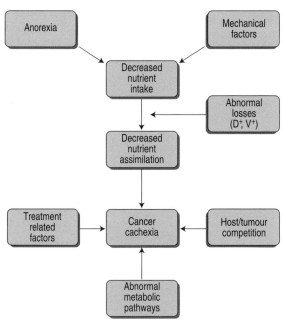

Figure 6.1   Diagram demonstrating effects that contribute towards cancer cachexia. D+, diarrhoea; V+, vomiting.

matter or ≤20% of metabolized energy. Providing metabolizable energy from fat is the most beneficial for the animal. Increased dietary fibre may aid in preventing abnormal stool quality (e.g. soft stools, or diarrhoea), which is commonly encountered when changing from a high-carbohydrate commercial dry food to a high-fat commercial or homemade diet. Recommendations of crude fibre levels greater than 2.5% dry matter base (DMB) are documented.[1]

Protein

Tumours use amino acids as a preferred source of energy. This results in an altered metabolism, with the patient having to increase skeletal protein breakdown, liver protein synthesis and whole body synthesis for tumour growth. This can become clinically significant when protein degradation exceeds intake. The immune response, wound healing rates and gastrointestinal functioning are also affected by the imbalances in protein levels. Specific amino acids have been shown to have different effects in cancer patients.

Arginine and glutamine are commonly supplemented in diets specifically designed for cancer patients. The addition of arginine to total parenteral nutrition (TPN) solutions can decrease tumour growth and metabolic rate in rodent models. In canine models quality of life and survival time have been increased when fed arginine in conjunction with n-3 fatty acids. Glutamine is also added to most human and veterinary enteral formulas. Glutamine has been shown to be beneficial in improving intestinal morphometry, reducing bacterial translocation, enhancing local immunity and improving survival times. Glutamine is a conditional essential amino acid. Supplementation is recommended when protein metabolism is altered, as in cancer patients.

The amino acids methionine and asparagine are both used in tumour cell growth. Methionine's precursor, homocysteine, when supplemented in the diet can stop tumour cell growth progression into different growth phases. This enables cell-cycle-specific therapeutic agents to target more tumour cells. Use of L-asparaginase in dogs and cats with lymphoma has high remission rates of 80%, due to asparagine being an essential factor in cell growth. The supplementation of glycine can also have important implications depending on the type of chemotherapy being utilized. Glycine will reduce cisplatin-induced nephrotoxicity.

Fats

A larger proportion of the metabolizable energy should be from dietary fat and oils. This is due to tumour cells having difficulty utilizing fats and oils. If cachexia is present an increase in dietary fat can improve the body condition scores. 25–40% on a dry matter basis is an ideal dietary fat content, or 50–65% of the calories on an 'as-fed basis'. Lipid metabolism also alters in cancer patients. Increased blood concentration of free fatty acids, very low density lipoproteins, triglycerides, plasma lipoproteins and hormone-dependent lipoprotein lipase activity can occur due to an overall decrease in lipogenesis and increased lipolysis. These changes in lipid metabolism can also cause immunosuppression, which relates to a decrease in survival time.

Omega-3 (n-3) fatty acids, like EPA and DHA, generally have an inhibiting effect on tumour growth. EPA can decrease protein degradation without altering protein synthesis, thus aiding in the symptoms associated with cachexia. The ratio of n-3 to n-6 fatty acids is important, as omega-6 (n-6) fatty acids such as linoleic and γ-linolenic acid enhance metastasis.

Vitamins and minerals

The levels of vitamins and minerals within the diet need to be sufficient to meet daily nutrient requirements. Higher levels of the antioxidant vitamins and minerals should be advocated in order to counteract damage caused by free radical action, and improve immune response. There are two hypotheses surrounding the use of antioxidants in cancer patients. The first supports the role of antioxidants within the diet, as they may improve the efficacy of cancer therapy by improving immune function, increasing tumour response to radiation or chemotherapy, decreasing toxicity to normal cells, and help to reverse metabolic changes contributing towards cachexia.[2] The second hypothesis states that antioxidants may have a deleterious effect by protecting cancer calls against damage by chemotherapy or radiation therapy.[2]

Serum levels of the trace minerals zinc, chromium and iron are lower in dogs with lymphoma and osteosarcoma than in healthy dogs.[3] Diets that are complete and balanced should not need supplementation of these trace minerals, although in homemade diets it should be considered.

Feeding a cancer diet

Initial assessment of the patient needs to be performed. Regular reassessments and calculations of daily energy requirements (DER) will be needed, especially if weight loss or cachexia starts to occur. If hospitalized, patients need to ingest at least their resting energy requirements (RER). At home, the calculated DER (RER × appropriate factor) is required. An initial illness factor of 1.25 in early stages of cancer, increasing to 1.75 in later stages has been recommended.

Because of the altered metabolic processes discussed, modifying nutrient intake is required. Several veterinary therapeutic diets are available, and with an increased fat content are very palatable. A suitable period of transition to the new diet is required. Some animals, however, can suffer diarrhoea due to the increase in fat content, and may need a longer period of transition.

With all cancer patients care should be taken with monitoring weight loss, especially in those that are initially overweight. Rapid weight loss, due to anorexia and alterations in metabolism, can result in a loss of lean muscle mass. Fat stores may still remain and may mask the detrimental effect of protein catabolism. Careful muscle condition scores and body condition scores will need to be performed, as 'overcoat syndrome' can quite easily be present.

The use of appetite stimulants can be useful in some cancer patients. The administration of diazepam or oxazepam is commonly used in practice, but can be unreliable in ensuring adequate calorie intake. In human cancer patients, megestrol acetate has been used to increase appetite and aid in weight gain. The benefits of this drug, in this situation, have not yet been determined in animals. If appetite stimulants fail and long-term nutritional support is required, enteral feeding techniques do need to be considered.

Key points

- Aim to prevent cancer cachexia.
- If the animal is unwilling to consume the cancer diet, inadequate calorific intake can result. It is best to feed anything, to ensure correct calorific intake.
- Quality of life for the animal is the most important factor.

Active encouragement to eat still needs to be initiated by the owner, or practice staff if hospitalized.

Support for the owner is greatly required with cancer patients. The word cancer will make any owner anxious, especially if the animal is anorexic, which can be very distressing. Many animals will be susceptible to this in their owners and it can be another factor associated with anorexia.

CASE STUDY 6.1

A 3-year-old Rottweiler was presented for examination by the owner who was concerned that the dog was suffering from a sudden onset of lameness of its left forelimb. On radiography a tumour (osteosarcoma) was discovered in the distal left radius. The dog was obese, and weighed 60 kg (ideal weight 50 kg). A weight-reduction programme (with prescription diets) for this dog at this stage is not currently advisable, as the leg was to be amputated and chemotherapy to be initiated. The dog was instead transferred to a light maintenance diet, and weight was lost. The dog was transferred to a prescription diet as target weight was reached. The diet did, however, induce diarrhoea in the dog. This can sometimes occur in animals that are used to consuming a diet with a higher fibre content. Close monitoring of weight was required in this case due to the higher fat content in the new diet.

References

1. Sheng-Long YE, Istafan NW, Driscoll DF. Tumour and host response to arginine and branch chain amino acid enriched total parenteral nutrition. Cancer 1992; 69:261–270.
2. Roudebush P, Davenport DJ, Novotny BJ. The use of nutraceuticals in cancer therapy. Vet Clin Small Anim 2004; 34:249–269.
3. Kazmierski KJ, Ogilvie GK, Fettman MJ, et al. Serum zinc, chromium and iron concentrations in dogs with lymphoma and osteosarcoma. J Vet Intern Med 2001; 15:585–588.

7

Cardiac disease

The nutritional status of the cardiac patient is exceptionally important to ascertain as it can have several effects on the animal. This can include the choice and dose rate of the drugs used in the medical treatment, interpretation of any laboratory results, interpretation of ECG data, prognosis of both surgical and medical intervention and the choice of diet for the patient. As part of the initial clinical assessment a full history of the animal's diet should be taken (Appendix 3). Nutrition can be a causative factor in cardiac disease. The factors associated with induced cardiac disease are the use of unusual supplements, not feeding a complete diet, or feeding a homemade or fad diet, and more than one animal in the household affected. Micro- and macronutrient deficiencies (calcium, potassium) can cause cardiac problems and thus a complete blood work-up needs to be performed.

Assessment of body condition and muscle scores of each individual animal is important with cardiac patients. A reduction in skeletal muscle mass might indicate energy malnutrition, and possibly a negative nitrogen balance. Animals with catabolic disease such as hyperthyroidism in cats, and cardiac failure lose body mass very rapidly, as with anorexic cats. The progression of cardiac disease can be exacerbated in obese animals. This can result in cardiomegaly, circulatory congestion, oedema, ascites and hypocalcaemia. An overweight animal must be objectively assessed; obesity must be differentiated from abdominal distension due to hepatomegaly or ascites. Obesity can also mask an underlying lean muscle body mass. Radiography can be useful in determining lack of lean body mass; this is especially notable on the proximal limbs. Obese animals need to lose weight in a controlled monitored way, the same as in a normal healthy animal. Obesity not only produces clinical signs (see Box 7.1) that mimic those of early heart failure, but can also cause cardiovascular changes that can exacerbate any underlying cardiovascular disease.

The aims of clinical nutrition are:

- to help control signs associated with sodium and fluid retention, by avoiding nutritional deficiencies and excesses
- to aid in maintaining normal heart muscle function
- to slow the progression of concurrent renal disease
- to support patients receiving diuretics or ACE inhibitors
- to maintain optimal weight, and aid in preventing cardiac cachexia.

Cardiac cachexia

34–75% of dogs with heart disease suffer from anorexia, and it is one of the multifactorial processes associated with the loss of lean body mass in cardiac cachexia.[1] Other factors include increased energy requirements and metabolic alterations. Cardiac

---

Box 7.1 Cardiovascular adaptations that occur during the transition from ideal body score to obese

- Increased perfusion requirements of expanding adipose tissue
- Elevated cardiac output
- Abnormal left ventricular function
- Variable blood pressure response (normotensive to hypertensive)
- Increased retention of sodium and water by the kidney
- Increased plasma aldosterone and norepinephrine (noradrenaline) concentration
- Increased left arterial pressure
- Increased heart rate
- Exercise intolerance

---

cachexia is more commonly seen in dogs than in cats, and in dilated cardiomyopathy (DCM) or right-sided heart failure. The primary energy source for animals with acute or chronic disease is amino acids from muscle, thus causing a reduction in lean body mass. Cachexia is a slow progressive process of the loss of lean body mass/muscle. Careful examination of obese animals is required, as this lean body mass reduction can occur, creating overcoat syndrome, and be easily missed. Any clinical nutrition of these animals includes management of any anorexia that is present.

Clinical nutrition

L-Carnitine

L-Carnitine is critical for fatty acid metabolism and energy production, and cardiac myocytes depend upon the oxidation of fatty acids for their energy. L-Carnitine deficiencies and a causative link with DCM have not been established, although deficiencies within the cardiac myocytes occur in 50% of dogs suffering with DCM. Some affected dogs with DCM do respond to L-carnitine supplementation. Supplementation of 50–100 mg/kg BW orally every 8 hours has been recommended for dogs with DCM,[1] though most cardiac diets are already supplemented with L-carnitine.

Fats

The role of fatty acids in the diet of cardiac patients has been widely reported. Supplementation of the diet with EPA and DHA has been shown to improve cachexia scores, thus improving quality of life, but had no effect on survival time. Animals suffering from cardiac cachexia have an increased production of inflammatory cytokines. These cytokines are directly linked to causing anorexia, to increased energy requirements and to increased catabolism of lean body mass.[1] Supplementation of the diet with omega-3 fatty acids (especially EPA and DHA) decreases the production and effects of cytokines.

Recommended dosage of 40 mg/kg BW of EPA and 25 mg/kg BW of DHA for both dogs and cats with anorexia or cachexia has been noted.[1] With most fish oil supplements containing 180 mg EPA and 120 mg of DHA per capsule, dosages can be easily calculated.[1]

Carbohydrates

The level of carbohydrates in the diet has to provide adequate calories for the specific lifestage. In the majority of cases this is for senior animals. The calorific value of the diet therefore tends to be of a lower level. It should also be remembered that these animals tend to have a more sedentary lifestyle due to the cardiac disease, and the risk for weight gain, or already being obese, is greater.

The recommended fibre levels in the diet are very much dependent on the individual. If the animal is obese, it is initially recommended that the animal reduces in weight and reaches its optimal bodyweight and body condition score (BCS). This may involve the use of a high-fibre diet. In animals that are already at an ideal BCS and optimal weight, fibre should be present but not excessive. The presence of fibre in the diet does reduce the bioavailability of many of the nutrients. As concurrent disease or impairment of the gastrointestinal tract, pancreas and liver can occur, a high–fibre diet is not ideal.[2]

Vitamins and minerals

The nutrients of main concern in patients with heart failure include sodium, potassium and magnesium. Treats and snacks that are often fed to dogs have a high salt content, as do cheese and processed meats, which are often used to administer medications. The restriction of sodium in the diet is useful in the mechanism to reduce fluid retention that accompanies many forms of heart disease. Both sodium and water can be retained when the rennin–angiotensin–aldosterone (RAA) cascade is stimulated, or when the patient's blood pressure falls.[3] One of the current methods of treatment for fluid retention is the use of diuretics. The diuretics block sodium retention but also promote urinary loss of magnesium and potassium. The prolonged use of diuretics can also lead to deficiencies of the water-soluble vitamins.

As a result of the cascade being stimulated extracellular and vascular fluid volume increase, thus increasing preload. The plasma protein concentration therefore becomes more dilute, which in turn decreases plasma oncotic pressure. Water moves from the vascular to the interstitial compartment resulting in oedema, ascites and congestion.

The use of angiotensin-converting enzyme (ACE) inhibitors has led to modification of the recommendation for sodium restriction in senior diets and early cardiac disease diets. ACE inhibitors are designed to block the production of angiotensin II and its subsequent stimulation of the secretion of aldosterone. Both of these chemicals promote retention of water and sodium by the kidney. Thus ACE inhibitors result in impaired sodium and water excretion. Sodium intake needs to be limited in proportion to the severity of the disease (see Table 7.1) in an attempt to avoid excesses. ACE inhibitors can also cause the retention of potassium; thus periodic serum levels should be monitored.[4] Spironolactone has similar potassium-sparing effects, along with being an aldosterone antagonist. Chronic renal failure (CRF) is often a concomitant disease of patients with cardiovascular disorders.

Table 7.1 Functional classification of heart failure and corresponding sodium intake

Class	Description[a]	Recommended upper limits of sodium intake (mg/kg BW/day)
I	Normal physical activity: symptoms not induced under normal exercise levels	Unrestricted
II	Slightly limited physical capacity: original physical activity leads to clinical signs	6.8
III	Markedly limited physical capacity: limited physical activity leads to clinical signs	4.5
IV	Unable to carry on any activity without signs: clinical signs present at rest	2.8

[a]Clinical signs include weight loss, exercise intolerance, coughing, respiratory distress and occasionally ascites.

Table 7.2 Comparison of feeding restricted sodium diets vs commercial diets with a high comparison sodium level

Food A	Food B	Preferring food A (%)	Preferring food B (%)	Number of animals
Canine h/d, dry	Purina Dog Chow	95	5	60
Canine h/d, dry	Iams Chunks	60	40	60
Canine h/d, dry	Pedigree Chum original	95	5	60
Canine h/d, canned	Ken-L-Ration Original	100	0	60

Diets for these animals also need restricted phosphorus levels. Levels of potassium and magnesium should also be optimally controlled as this supports the patient receiving diuretics and/or ACE inhibitor therapy.

Magnesium levels can have a deleterious effect on a range of cardiovascular conditions including hypertension, congestive heart failure, coronary artery disease and cardiac arrhythmias.[4] Hypomagnesaemia can be induced through the use of digoxin and loop diuretics.

The B vitamin complex is often supplemented in cardiac diets. At present there has been little investigation into the role of vitamin B deficiency as a cause of heart disease in dogs and cats. Polyuria and anorexia can both contribute to low vitamin B concentrations, and thus vitamin B requirements are higher.

Recommendations of higher levels of antioxidants in animals suffering from CHF are commonplace, owing to the by-product reactive oxygen species (ROS). Coenzyme Q_{10}, another antioxidant, has also been anecdotally recommended. Coenzyme Q_{10}, like L-carnitine, is a cofactor in a number of energy-producing reactions. Benefits of supplementation include improved myocardial metabolic efficiency and increases in antioxidant production.[1] Although no direct evidence has been obtained in establishing coenzyme Q_{10}'s direct benefits, recommended dosages of 30 mg orally twice a day (b.i.d.), and in large breeds of dog up to 90 mg orally b.i.d., have been reported.[1]

Proteins

Taurine is an essential amino acid in cats, because it is the only amino acid able to combine with cholesterol during bile salt synthesis, whereas in other species another amino acid, glycine, can be substituted. Cats do have a limited ability to synthesise taurine from cysteine and methionine, but its use outstrips production. The mechanism of heart failure in cats and dogs with taurine deficiency is poorly understood. Prior to 1987 supplementation of commercial foods with taurine was not commonplace and the number of cases of feline DCM was large. Clinical studies have also shown that inadequate potassium intake may be sufficient to induce a significant taurine depletion and cardiovascular disease in cats. Most dogs presenting with DCM do not tend to have a concurrent taurine deficiency, although in some breeds where DCM is not a common disease, a taurine deficiency has been noted. Dog breeds reported to be associated with taurine deficiency include the American cocker spaniel, golden retriever, Labrador, Newfoundland, Dalmatian and English bulldog.[1]

The overall protein level in the diet is reduced. This is due to the progression of renal disease, which is associated with cardiac disease. The protein levels are therefore restricted but of a high biological value; typical values of 17% dry matter base (DMB) for dogs and 29% (DMB) for cats are often recommended.

It should be noted that if protein is too restricted this can be detrimental to the animal. Protein malnutrition can rapidly occur in the presence of catabolic disease and inadequate food intake. Hypoproteinaemia can be present in cardiac disease with reduced liver function. In animals with cardiac cachexia, protein levels should be increased. Supplementing a cardiac diet with scrambled eggs or cottage cheese is an excellent method of increasing the protein levels without increasing the salt content of the diet.

Feeding the cardiac patient

Each diet must be based around each individual's specific requirements. Overweight or obese animals will require diets aimed at calorie restriction. Underweight patients require a calorie-dense diet. Concurrent disease also needs to be taken into consideration. Laboratory parameters should be obtained to identify any electrolyte excesses or deficiencies. Anorexia is a common side effect of CHF, and great effort on behalf of the owner may be required in order to entice the animal to eat.

Feeding a low-salt diet

Low-salt diets are used for both cardiac and renal patients. It is often a misconception that low-salt diets have a reduced palatability. Studies have demonstrated that diets with reduced sodium chloride levels used in patients with cardiovascular disease have comparable or better palatability than supermarket brands (see Table 7.2).[5] Difficulties in transition from the patient's original diet to a low-salt prescription diet can be attributed to:

- advanced illness associated with renal and heart failure
- established eating and feeding habits of both the animal and the owner
- anorexia associated with disease process and/or medications
- too quick a transition and/or established food aversions.

Transition to a low-salt diet is always easier if the animal has already been fed a diet in a lower-salt category. Animals are often encouraged to consume a new diet by adding flavour enhancers. Low-sodium additives can include low-sodium soups and sweeteners, such as honey or syrups. Table 7.3 demonstrates how adding certain foodstuffs to the diet can significantly increase the sodium intake. As with all clinical prescription diets, the therapeutic agent of the diet should not be imposed if it is detrimental to the overall nutrient intake. Owners should be aware that both trial and error might be required in these

Table 7.3 Daily sodium intake for a dog and cat eating various foods: based on a 15 kg dog consuming 935 kcal/day, and a 4 kg cat consuming 270 kcal/day

Food	Sodium intake (mg/day)
Dog	
Grocery moist diet	2845
Grocery dry diet	1144
Senior dry diet	390
Renal moist diet	400
Cardiac dry diet	111
30 g cheese	262
1 slice of bread	218
Cat	
Grocery moist diet	952
Grocery dry food	371
Senior dry diet	186
Renal/cardiac moist diet	175
Renal/cardiac dry diet	156
½ tin tuna	160

patients. Some animals can 'go off' certain diets and a cyclical approach with two or three commercial diets may be required. Use of different feeding methods along with different foods should be utilized. The success of a transition to a new diet does hugely depend on the dedication of the owner and the support received by the veterinary practice. Supporting the owner can be achieved by providing a list of foodstuffs and their sodium content. If the animal is overweight or underweight then a weight-management programme must be initiated.

Administering medications can be difficult, and many of the foods used to 'hide' medications can be high in salt. Advising owners on different methods can aid in an increase in compliance. Alternatives can include:

- Teaching the owner to administer medications without the use of foods. This can include the use of pill givers.

- The use of commercial treats designed to hold medications. Always double-check the salt content.
- Use of appropriate foods such as bananas (good potassium source), no-added-salt peanut butter (not ideal in obese animals), and home-cooked meats (without added salt), not sandwich/processed meats.

Key points

- Ensure that the daily calorie and nutrient intake is met.
- The optimal BCS needs to be achieved in both obese and underweight animals.
- Restrict sodium intake.

References

1. Freeman LM, Rush JE. Nutritional modulation of heart disease. In: Ettinger SJ, Feldman EC, eds. Textbook of veterinary internal medicine. Volume 1. 6th edn. St Louis, Missouri: Elsevier Saunders; 2005.
2. Roudebush P. Study cited in Roudebush P, Keene BW, Mizelle L. Cardiovascular disease. In: Hand MS, Thatcher CD, Remillard RL, et al., eds. Small animal clinical nutrition. 4th edn. Missouri: Mark Morris Institute; 2000:529–562.
3. Davies M. Feeding the cardiac patient. In: Kelly N, Wills J, eds. BSAVA Manual of companion animal nutrition and feeding. Gloucester: BSAVA Publications; 1996:117–127.
4. Buffington CAT, Holloway C, Abood SK. Manual of veterinary dietetics. St Louis, Missouri: Elsevier Saunders; 2004
5. Roudebush P, Keene BW, Mizelle L. Cardiovascular disease. In: Hand MS, Thatcher CD, Remillard RL, et al., eds. Small animal clinical nutrition. 4th edn. Missouri: Mark Morris Institute; 2000:529–562.

8
Critical care nutrition

With all sick companion animals the nutritional goal is for the patient to eat the designated diet in its own environment. Unfortunately in critically sick animals they will be in a hospital environment, where the added stress of this different environment can affect food consumption. Most animals will require, or benefit from, a veterinary therapeutic diet, but the initial goal is to ensure that the patient is receiving its daily calorific requirement. Analgesia should not be forgotten, as pain can reduce food intake in some animals. Hydration status must be maintained and corrected before any nutritional support can be initiated (Fig. 8.1). The aim of critical care nutrition is dependent on the disease process and/or the individual's specific requirements. Each case must be considered in terms of its own specific requirements once a full clinical examination and history has been achieved. This includes nutritional assessment and dietary history. The sole aim can be defined as to prevent and/or treat malnutrition when present. In order to define any nutritional aims in more depth, it is more beneficial to split the aims into short-term and long-term goals. The short-term aims are to:

- provide for any ongoing nutritional requirements (both in terms of energy and nutrients)
- prevent or correct any nutritional deficiencies or imbalances
- minimize metabolic derangements
- prevent further catabolism of lean body mass.

Long-term nutritional aims should include:

- restoration of optimal body condition
- provision of required nutrients to the animal within its own environment.

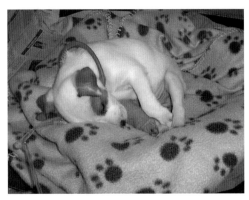

Figure 8.1   Critically ill cases require hydration levels to be maintained at all times.

As disease processes change, and the animal's physiological and metabolic responses alter, the nature of the nutritional support, and both the short-term and long-term nutritional aims may alter.

When assessing animals for the preferred method of critical care feeding the nutritional status of the animal needs to be evaluated. This should include body conditions score (BCS), muscle conditions score (MCS), hydration status, weight, hair coat quality, signs of inadequate wound healing, hypoalbuminaemia, lymphopenia and coagulopathy.[1] Thought should be given to 'fluid shifts' in these animals, as they can severely affect haematological values and the animal's weight. Factors that should be identified include specific electrolyte imbalances, hyperglycaemia, hypertriglyceridaemia or hyperammonaemia, as they will have large consequences on the nutritional critical care plan. Adequate adjustments will be required to the feeding plan and possibly the formulation of any parenteral nutrition to be utilized.

The calorific intake required by the patient depends on several factors:

- the rate of energy use for basal metabolism (resting)
- nutrient assimilation
- body temperature maintenance
- activity levels.

Energy requirements during sickness are based on resting energy requirements (RER). This is due to the assumption that the patient is inactive and is often confined to a small area. Because of this, calculated energy requirements using an illness factor are only a guideline (Table 8.1). Daily weighing of the patient, assessing healing rates and assessing lean body mass are good indicators of whether the patient is receiving sufficient calories. In herbivores (horses and rabbits) vital parameters should also include gastrointestinal mobility, and faecal volume, appearance and frequency should be monitored. In the early phases of supportive feeding, digital pulses in equines should be monitored. This is due to the potential to induce carbohydrate-induced laminitis.

As with all hospitalized patients, human and animal, malnutrition has been associated with an increase in infectious morbidity, prolonged hospital stay and an increase in mortality. The recommendations of nutritional management of sick horses have been constructed from extrapolated data from other species. There have been no controlled studies on the relationship between nutritional support and clinically important endpoints, such as surgical complication rates, duration of hospitalized period and mortality rates in this species.

The volume of liquid diets administered at each bolus feeding in dogs and cats should not exceed 50 ml/kg. This is only an estimate and each animal should be judged on an individual basis. Tolerance to liquid diets is best when small feeds are delivered frequently. In horses a reasonable target is to feed 2–4 l every 2–4 hours. Once these volumes are well

Table 8.1   **Illness factors when calculating resting energy requirements (RER) for sick dogs and cats**

Burns:	
Moderate	RER × 1.5
Severe	RER × 2.0
Cage rest	RER × 1.25
Cancer:	
Early	RER × 1.25
Late	RER × 1.75
Sepsis	RER × 1.7–1.8
Surgery or trauma:	
Mild	RER × 1.3–1.6
Severe	RER × 1.5–1.7

tolerated, the volume of food in each meal can be increased with the frequency decreased. A 500 kg horse has an average stomach capacity of 7–9 l, but no single feed should exceed 6 l.[2]

Starvation and anorexia

Starvation can leave the animal severely emaciated, but also the gastrointestinal tract will become atrophied, due to the inadequate nutrient supply. Intestinal villi become atrophied and the epithelial layers become thin and fragile. Bacterial translocation will often occur in these cases. The gastrointestinal capacity to digest and absorb nutrients will become severely limited. The loss of lean body mass occurs from skeletal muscle and internal tissues. Nutritional support of these animals is vital and required immediately. Initially, hydration, electrolytes and acid–base status of the patient need to be rectified. The diet chosen needs to be of a high digestibility, and primarily consisting of proteins and fats. This is due to the patient utilizing these nutrients over carbohydrates. The patient will be suffering from protein energy malnutrition (PEM) and the quality of the protein feed is important. On initiating nutritional support to the patient, small frequent meals are required, slowly building up over a period of time to the full daily nutrient and energy requirements. PEM has a potential to occur during times of illness and when increased demands for protein and energy are made.[3]

Transient diarrhoea is a common side effect in these cases because of maldigestion, and should resolve as the patient recovers. Inclusion of dietary fibre in the diet should be avoided, as it will reduce the digestibility of the diet and bind nutrients that are required.

Clinical nutrition

Water (hydration levels)
The initial stage of nutritional support is correcting any dehydration, electrolyte replacement and normalization of the acid–base status before starting assisted feeding. Initiating assisted feeding before the patient is haemodynamically stable can further compromise the patient. If oedema occurs or dehydration persists, recalculation of flow rates is required.

Monitoring of hydration level indicators is required during intravenous fluid therapy (see Table 2.1 and Box 2.1, p. 14). Daily maintenance fluid requirements are approximately 50–60 ml/kg BW/day, or 2 ml/kg BW/hour. If persistent vomiting or diarrhoea is present these additional losses need to be factored in.

Where dogs and cats are able to consume fluids without vomiting, the use of an oral rehydration fluid should be advocated. Unless contraindicated, a bowl or bucket of water should be placed in the animal's kennel or stable. If required, additional fluids can always be administered intravenously, or via feeding tubes.

Protein
Protein energy malnutrition (PEM) can occur during periods of illness, injury or even after routine operations. During these periods the body shuts down systems in order to conserve the limited resources. Physiological changes such as a drop in blood pressure, reduction in cardiac output and a drop in oxygen consumption occur. This is clinical shock and is known as the ebb phase. Clinical shock is treatable but the length of time that shock is suffered is variable, and can ultimately be lethal. Following the ebb phase is the flow or hypermetabolic phase. During this second phase the patient's body defence and repair mechanisms are initiated. This process is where anorexia and starvation differ.[4]

Nutritional support with adequate protein levels is vital; patients in a catabolic state will utilize the skeletal muscle proteins. Sufficient calories need to be supplied to the patient from fats and carbohydrates. This will ensure that proteins are not used as a source of energy. The quality of the proteins provided is of importance as is the digestibility. Specific amino acids are supplemented to critical care diets. Glutamine is an important substrate for the increased levels of gluconeogenesis occurring in rapidly dividing cells. Any deficiency in this amino acid has been shown to lead to gut mucosal atrophy and an increase in bacterial translocation, due to a compromise of the mucosal barrier. This has led to the suggestion that glutamine may behave as a 'conditionally essential' amino acid during severe illness. The essential amino acid arginine has a positive effect on the immune system and can subsequently improve survival times of septic patients. Many enteral diets are supplemented with both glutamine and arginine. High doses of glutamine have a trophic effect on the gut mucosa.

The use of a novel protein source in these cases has been advocated. Because of the atrophy of the gastrointestinal tract, protein antigens can cross through to the bloodstream and set up hypersensitivity processes.

Vitamins and minerals

The supplementation of vitamins and minerals for hospitalized patients will depend on the disease and its severity. Sodium, chloride, potassium, phosphate, calcium and magnesium should be used for short-term nutritional support. All animals that receive intravenous fluid therapy, with or without parenteral support, should have daily electrolyte levels monitored. If any polydipsia or polyuria is present, supplementation of the water-soluble vitamins is required. Zinc aids in promoting wound healing and plays a role in protein and nucleic acid metabolism. Supplementation of nutritional support diets with zinc has been recommended.

Carbohydrates

Carbohydrates within any critical care diet need to be of a very high digestibility. The quantities of fibre need to be kept to a minimum, as it will decrease digestibility and bind up important nutrients. The level of carbohydrate in the diet needs to be sufficient to supply the required calories for recovery.

Fats

The quantity of fat in a critical care diet needs to be increased. A higher level of calories can be obtained from fat rather than via carbohydrates. The inclusion of omega-3 fatty acids can help decrease any inflammatory response.

Rabbit critical care nutrition

Rabbits need prompt treatment when anorexia presents; this is especially important in obese rabbits and pregnant or lactating does. This is due to the greater risk of developing hepatic lipidosis and/or other clinical disorders.[5] Table 8.2 sets out to

Table 8.2 Relevant clinical signs and/or history in the anorexic rabbit[5]

Clinical sign and/or history	Significance
History of a stressful event	Predisposes to GI hypomotility
Poor diet	Predisposes to GI hypomotility and dental disease
Sudden onset of profound anorexia and depression	Abdominal catastrophe (e.g. intestinal obstruction)
Weight loss	Suggests a chronic problem, e.g. dental disease, CRF, neoplasia or GI hypomotility
Ataxia	Locomotor or neurological disease. Can also occur in the later stages of GI hypomotility and hepatic lipidosis
Absence of faeces	Disruption in the normal digestive function
Diarrhoea	Enteritis, enterotoxaemia, antibiotic associated D+, or coccidiosis
Depression	Associated with abdominal pain
Abdominal discomfort	Suggests abdominal disease, e.g. gastric dilation, intestinal obstruction
Problems with mastication	Dental disease
Salivation	Dental disease
Soiled perineum	An indication of ill health, can be due to pain, dental problems, urinary tract disease, lack of fibre in the diet, or loss of flexibility due to obesity or spondylosis

GI, gastrointestinal; CRF, chronic renal failure; D+, diarrhoea describe some of the more common clinical signs associated with anorexia, and their possible causes.

Syringe feeding must be initiated in rabbits that have not eaten for more than 24 hours. A nasogastric tube is rarely used, but is ideal. Rabbits get stressed in unfamiliar environments; illness, anorexia and syringe feeding exacerbate this. The nasogastric tube should be used more as it reduces stress levels, whilst maintaining gastrointestinal tract (GIT) health and providing the required nutrients for the rabbit. Several preparations are available on the market for critical care nutrition for rabbits, and it is important that they contain both soluble and insoluble fibre sources. Fresh grass and other foods should be made available to the rabbit at all times, even when not eating. Provision of alfalfa to rabbits recovering from major surgery or severe illness is recommended. Alfalfa tends to be very appealing to the rabbit's taste buds and will promote weight gain.

Analgesia should be routinely used. Pain will prevent the rabbit from eating and as a consequence reduced nutrient intake can occur. GIT motility stimulants such as cisapride (0.5 mg/kg BW) and metoclopramide (0.5 mg/kg BW) can be used in order to aid in the prevention of GI hypomotility in high-risk stimulations (e.g. after surgery).[5]

Equine critical care nutrition

Horses have good reserves of nutrients, and can tolerate 1–2 days of complete food deprivation (but not water deprivation). When repeated administration of fluids and supportive nutrition is required, the use of indwelling nasogastric tubes is fairly well tolerated in the short term. Indwelling tubes can be sutured to the nares or taped to the halter with the end positioned in the distal oesophagus or stomach. Repeated stomach tubing over a period of time can become stressful in any animal, and for longer periods oesophageal tubes should be considered. Complications of cellulitis and stricture formation can result. All tubes must be sealed between feedings in order to prevent aerophagia.

The procedure for placing feeding tubes is the same as that used for small animals. A high-protein gruel/slurry can be used (Table 8.3).[6]

Table 8.3 **Horse high-protein gruel/slurry required for tube feeding a 500 kg horse[a]**

Constituent	Amount	Comment
Water	20–24 l	This approximates to 5% bodyweight, and should be gradually increased over 7 days
Dextrose	300–900 g	Gradually increased over 7 days
Casein (or dehydrated cottage cheese)	300–900 g	Gradually increased over 7 days
Dehydrated alfalfa meal	1800–2000 g	Addition of this fibre source aids in reduction of diarrhoea. On rehydration it will expand, so add to the gruel mixture last
Electrolyte mixture:	Total of 230 g consisting of:	This electrolyte mixture will provide a high-potassium and low-sodium content to the gruel/slurry
NaCl	10 g	
$NaHCO_3$	15 g	
KCl	75 g	
K_2HPO_4	60 g	
$CaCl_2$ $2H_2O$	45 g	
MgO	25 g	

[a]It is recommended that this daily amount is divided into equal portions of three to four meals.

When feeding sick horses it is important to remember that the gastrointestinal flora is disrupted. Production of vitamins (especially vitamin B complexes) can become reduced and almost diminished. Supplementation of these vitamins is recommended.

Supportive feeding methods

Supportive feeding methods should be considered when there is a history of greater than 10% weight loss; decreased food intake; anorexia; increased nutrient demands due to trauma or surgery; increased nutrient losses resulting from vomiting, diarrhoea, burns or scalds; acute exacerbation of chronic disease; and if specific areas of the alimentary canal need to be bypassed. The ideal diet to use in these cases should be highly palatable, digestible and have a high energy density (Box 8.1). A relatively high percentage of energy should be provided as protein and fat rather than carbohydrates. Table 8.4 gives suggested levels of nutrients in critical care diets for cats and dogs. These diets are available in three different forms: powdered, liquid and moist diets. Moist diets can have thixotropic

Table 8.4 **Macronutrient levels in critical care diets (as % energy content of diet)**

	Protein	Fat	Carbohydrate
Dog	20–25	50–55	25–26
Cat	25–37	41–50	22–25

properties – when mixed their viscosity decreases, making them thinner.

The use of assisted feeding methods does have great advantages, but care of the feeding tube is vital. The artificial opening through the abdomen into the gastrointestinal tract through which the tube is inserted is referred to as a stoma. The stoma must be treated as a surgical wound, and cleaned daily with normal saline, or cooled boiled water, for the first 7–14 days, or until it is healed. Dressings around tubes are not always necessary, unless indicated, e.g. if the stoma site is infected, the animal is interfering with the insertion site. Table 8.5 lists some example problems that can arise with tube feeding. Deciding on which method of tube feeding to be utilized depends on a number of different factors. Figure 8.2 shows a simple flow chart with deciding factors.[7]

Encouraging animals to eat
The process of encouraging animals to eat should never be forgotten. Voluntary intake can be established in a number of cases by taking time out to personally encourage the animal to eat. Grooming can actively encourage the animals (especially dogs and cats) to eat, removing any nasal discharge that is blocking their sense of smell, as can tender loving care, providing competition, hand feeding, providing a selection of different diets, taking the animal into a different environment, and in some cases offering the animal some of the food that you are eating if it is suitable. This last method works especially well in dogs.

Syringe feeding
Many patients will tolerate syringe feeding well, as long as stress is limited during the process. Aversions can be initiated if the animal resents the process, and the food is forcibly fed. 50 ml catheter-tipped syringes (Figs 8. 3 and 8.4) or Pasteur pipettes (cut

---

Box 8.1   Calculations of enteral feeding amounts

1. Calculate the RER of the animal:

   RER = 70 × (BW kg)$^{0.75}$ for animals < 2 kg

   or > 45 kg, or 30 × (BW kg) + 70

2. Add in the illnesses factor:

   RER × Illness factor = kcal/day

3. Choose the specific diet that is most beneficial for the patient and the method of feeding.

4. Divide the energy content of the diet (kcal/ml or gram) by the energy requirement of the animal (kcal/day) to achieve the daily amount of food required.

5. Divide the total amount to be given in a day by the total number of feeds wished to be given, or by the maximum volume of each feed.

Table 8.5 Problems that can arise when utilizing tube feeding

Problem	Common causes	Signs and clinical symptoms	Treatment
Infection	Poor hygiene, contamination of the tube site by oral flora at the time of tube insertion	Inflammation, malodour, pain, increased exudates	Swab the site for culture and sensitivity, administer appropriate antibiotics. Apply dressings if indicated
Leakage	Poorly designed tube, infection, and over-granulation	Excessive movement of the tube or the tube cannot be moved, inflammation of the skin and/or excoriation	Identify the cause of the problem. Use a barrier cream around the tube insertion site
Over-granulation	Infection, incorrect positioning of the tube, excessive movement of the tube	Inflamed, red raised tissue, bleeding, pain	Treatment of any infection, correct any positioning problems
Blocked tube	Inadequate flushing regimen, damaged tube, medication interaction	Difficulty flushing tube, unable to administer water, feeds or medications	Review flushing regimen, possibly medications. Flush with soda water or enzymatic solution. Preparations used in human medicine use commercially prepared enzymes, e.g. Clog Zapper to remove blockages
Feed-associated problems such as poor tolerance	Feed rate, technique, method, timing of feeds or medications, or type of nutrition used	Bloating, nausea, vomiting, diarrhoea, constipation	Eliminate other causes. Review all feeding and medication regimens. Use a diet with a slightly higher fibre content
Aspiration	Incorrect positioning of the tube when feeding, feed rate/volume too high, poor gastric emptying	Chest infection, aspiration pneumonia, coughing, regurgitation of the feed	Review feed rate and administration method. Confirm that tube has been placed correctly, e.g. with radiography

down) are exceptionally useful in administering critical care diets.

Naso-oesophageal tubes

Naso-oesophageal tubes (Fig. 8.5) are generally well tolerated by cats and dogs and are suitable for short-term nutritional support, usually 3–7 days, though longer periods have been documented. Contraindications for the use of these tubes include unconsciousness, vomiting, disease or dysfunction of the pharynx, larynx and nares, swallowing reflex, oesophagus and stomach. The preferred placement of the naso-oesophageal tube is in the caudal oesophagus, rather than the stomach, as it reduces the risk of reflux oesophagitis.

Once the tube has been placed (Fig. 8.6), a small amount of water is injected slowly into the tube to see if a cough reflex is induced, indicating aspira-

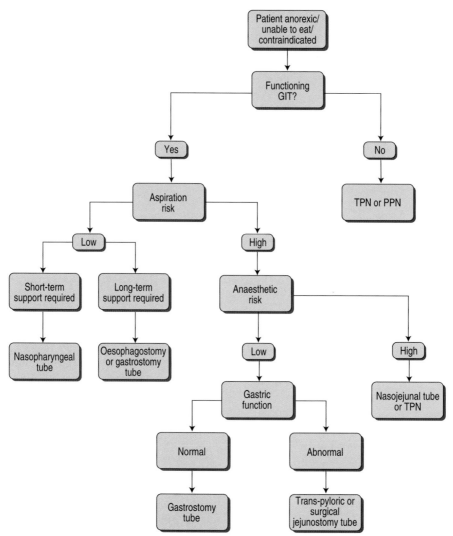

Figure 8.2 Flow diagram of assisted feeding decisions.[7] GIT, gastrointestinal tract; TPN, total parenteral nutrition; PPN, partial/peripheral parenteral nutrition.

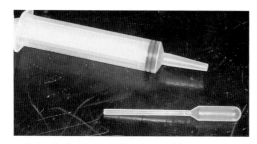

Figure 8.3 Syringe and pipette used for syringe feeding.

tion. Lateral radiographs can also identify that the tube has been correctly placed. Because of the narrow bore of the tube, blockages do occur. Injection of 5–10 ml of water into the tube following administration of the liquid diet, should aid in prevention of any blockages. If blockages do occur small amounts of carbonated drinks, cranberry juice or solutions of pancreatic enzymes have been shown to aid in their removal. Pre-feeding administration of water is required to ensure that the tube is still positioned correctly. In human medicine, preparations of 'Clog Zapper' are commonly used, and they can also be utilized in veterinary situations.[8]

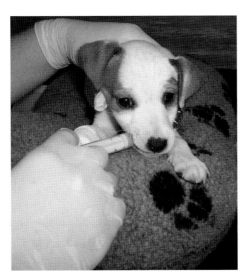

Figure 8.4 Syringe feeding puppy.

Pharyngostomy tubes
Pharyngostomy tubes (Figs 8.7 and 8.8) are commonly used in cats that have suffered facial trauma, usually after a road traffic accident. Pharyngostomy

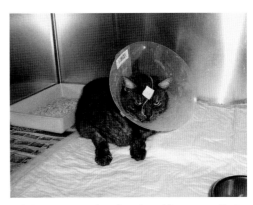

Figure 8.6 Nasogastric tube placed in a cat suffering from a fractured mandible.

tubes are of use when bypassing of the nose and mouth is required in order to administer nutritional support. Animals that do not tolerate naso-oesophageal tubes well can have pharyngostomy tubes placed. These types of tubes have been largely replaced by oesophagostomy tubes or gastrostomy tubes that are placed percutaneously.[9] Aseptic placement of the tube under general anaesthetic

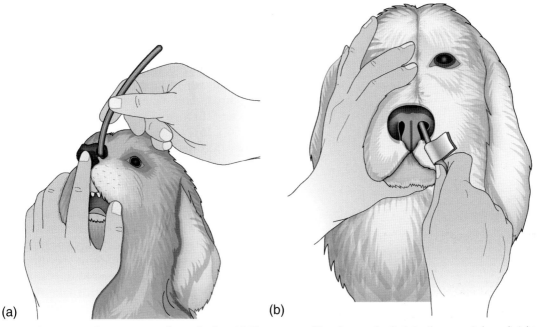

(a) (b)

Figure 8.5 Placement of a naso-oesophageal tube. (a) Placement of local anaesthetic into the nose is beneficial to the animal. Once the anaesthetic is working, the external nares are pushed dorsally and the tube is gently passed into the ventral nasal meatus. (b) The tube is fully inserted until the pen mark or adhesive tape tabs are reached. Glue or sutures are then used in order to secure the tube in position. It is, however, useful to check correct placement of the tube prior to securing it in place.

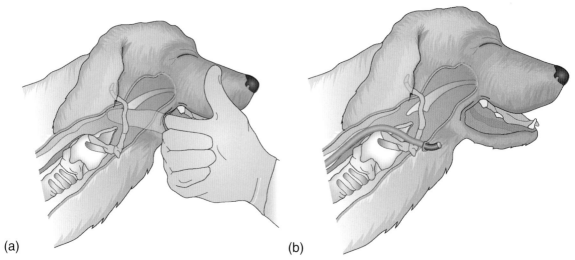

(a)   (b)

Figure 8.7 Placement of a pharyngostomy tube. (a) In order to correctly position the tube, a finger is used to pal-pate the hyoid apparatus of the anaesthetized animal. The tube exit needs to be as far caudally and dorsally along the pharyngeal wall as possible. Once an optimal site has been located, a 1-cm skin incision is made over the bulging pharyngeal wall. Blunt dissection is advocated in order to tunnel caudally through the tissues from outside to inside. (b) Forceps are used to grasp one end of the tube, whilst the other end is passed down the oesophagus. The tube is secured in place with tape and sutures.

is required. Frequent cleaning and inspection of the tube is necessary under aseptic conditions. Complications can include airway obstruction, damage to the cervical nerves and blood vessels, and infections.

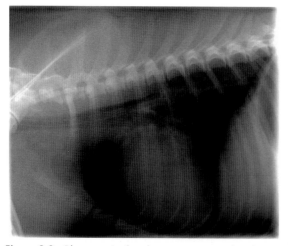

Figure 8.8 Placement of a pharyngostomy tube. An X-ray proves that the tube is not long enough, not reaching the caudal oesophagus. (Courtesy of K Lenton, The Veterinary Hospital Group, Plymouth.)

Percutaneous endoscopic gastrostomy (PEG) tubes

These tubes (Fig. 8.9) require placement under general anaesthetic, and need to be in place for at least 5 days prior to removal. PEG tubes are utilized when long-term nutritional support is required, and when oesophageal problems are present. In many cases of gastric dilation/volvulus (GDV), PEG tubes are placed at the time of gastropexy.[10] Adhesions between the gastric serosa and the peritoneum can form within 48–72 hours.[9] It should be noted that in malnourished patients these adhesions might take longer to form. Once the tube is placed (Fig. 8.10), only a third of the calculated daily energy requirements should be administered; then on day 2, two-thirds; and by the third day the full amount. Feeding through the PEG tube can commence 4 hours after its insertion. If patients are unable to take fluids orally, mouth care should be encouraged at least every 4 hours. This involves ensuring that the mucous membranes remain moist, and that bacterial infections are prevented. This can be managed by the use of oral hygiene gels that contain chlorohexidine designed for dental care.

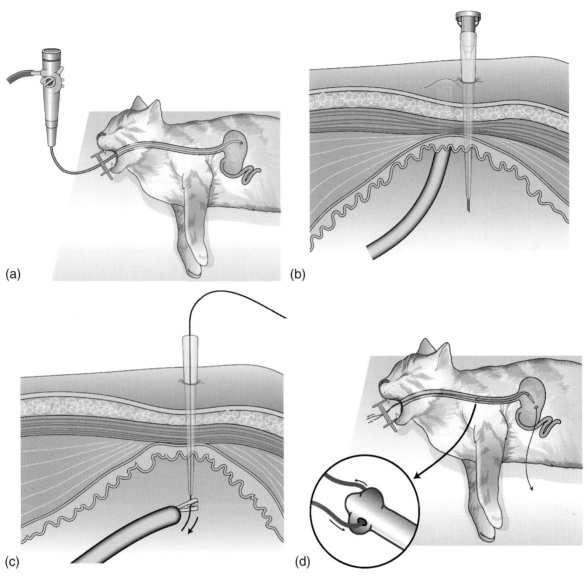

Figure 8.9 Placement of a PEG tube. (a) The animal should be placed in right lateral recumbency. The stomach is then insufflated with air introduced by the endoscope. The gastric wall will then become in contact with the body wall. (b) The lighted tip of the endoscope can be seen when pressed against the abdominal wall. This area should be prepared and scrubbed aseptically. A large-bore needle or over-the-needle catheter is inserted into the stomach next to the endoscope tip. (c) A thick nylon suture is fed through the needle or catheter, and is grasped by the endoscope's retrieval forceps. As the endoscope is withdrawn, the nylon suture is pulled out through the mouth. (d) The next stage is dependent on the type of tube used. In order to allow the feeding tube to be pulled through the abdominal wall a catheter needs to be threaded on to the drawn-through nylon prior to the feeding tube being attached. Some commercial kits (e.g. Pezzer catheter assembly kits) already have a catheter guide in place. The lubricated catheter (with attached feeding tube) is drawn down the oesophagus into the stomach by the suture which is exiting the body wall. (e) When the lubricated catheter guide reaches the body wall, resistance will be felt. Firm application of counter-pressure to the body wall should allow the catheter tip to emerge through the skin. In order for the feeding tube to exit, a very small incision (2–3 mm) may be required. (f) As the feeding tube is pulled through, gentle traction will be required in order to bring the stomach and abdominal wall into close contact. A rubber flange is then slid down the tube, and secured in place.

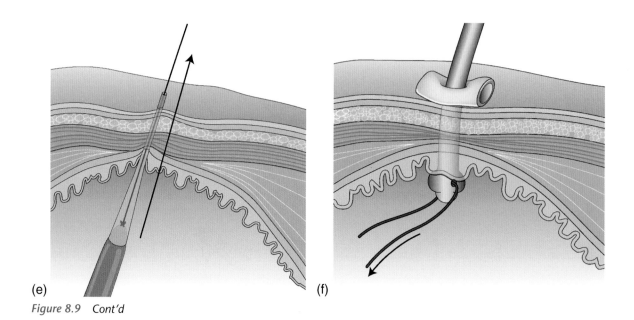

(e)   (f)

Figure 8.9 Cont'd

The procedure for removal of the gastrostomy tube in animals over 10 kg is to cut the catheter off flush with the skin after pulling it taught. The catheter tip is then passed in the faeces. The resulting gastrocutaneous fistula will rapidly heal if kept clean.

Microenteral nutrition

Microenteral nutrition is the delivery of very small amounts of water, electrolytes and easily absorbable nutrients directly into the GIT. This method is often underused in veterinary practices, but allows the nutritional requirements of the intestinal mucosa to be met. This helps to preserve the intestinal blood flow, the mucosal barrier and its immune function.[2] Initial volumes of 0.05–0.2 ml/kg BW/hour are recommended, and will add exceptionally little to the volume of fluids normally produced by the stomach. Gradual increases can occur to 1–2 ml/kg BW/hour, over a 24- to 48-hour period. Enteral solutions that can be used include oral rehydrating solutions, and those containing glutamine.

Parenteral nutrition

Parenteral nutrition (PN) is often fraught with complications, but should be considered in animals that are unable to tolerate enteral supportive feeding methods. This includes animals that are vomiting or regurgitating, or those unable to protect their airway. Complications such as hyperalimentation or overfeeding can be common, and lead to metabolic complications,[1] though these can be resolved easily by discontinuing, and respond fairly rapidly. Other complications can be more severe, and include localized infections, which can lead to septicaemia. The use of total parenteral nutrition (TPN) in equines can be limited due to the expense of maintaining fluids over a period of time. The use of a central line (in TPN cases) for administering supportive nutri-

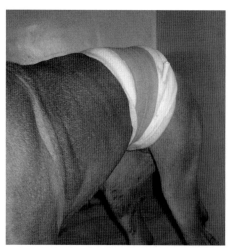

Figure 8.10 Correct bandaging of PEG tube in place.

tion requires careful attention to aseptic techniques. The PN solution can also act as the perfect reservoir for bacterial growth. In many cases of postoperative colic, the animal is usually toxic and very prone to jugular thrombosis; TPN can exacerbate this problem. Hence, thoracic, cephalic and saphenous veins are used, in order to preserve the jugular.

Parenteral nutrition can be divided into two different categories:

1. TPN – where parenteral nutrition is formulated to meet 100% of the animal's energy requirements. In all animals receiving TPN, hyperglycaemia and glucosuria can develop in some cases. This hyperglycaemic state possibly reflects the decrease in peripheral glucose uptake resulting from mild insulin resistance. This can precipitate laminitis in horses. As a general rule, intravenous (i.v.) dextrose solution should be used as the sole source of nutrition for no more than 2–3 days. An amino acid solution should be added to the dextrose solution, and then lipids. On day 1 of the administration ~12% of the animal's total fluid requirement should be given; on day 2 ~24%. The remainder of the fluids should be administered as i.v. fluids. An example of a TPN solution will contain 32% lipid energy, 9% protein energy and 60% carbohydrate energy.

2. Partial parenteral nutrition (PPN) – formulated to meet 40–70% of the animal's total energy requirements. These solutions are diluted, which decreases the protein and caloric density, but allows the solution to be administered via peripheral veins. Peripheral PN can also be used to describe PPN.[1] A lower osmolarity of solution is required, and this is achieved by using 5% dextrose preparations rather than 50%. PPN is only intended for short-term use (less than 5 days), and should be limited to animals that are not debilitated. It should be noted that purely dextrose solutions are not appropriate for the long-term treatment of hypoglycaemia. In critical care situations insulin resistance and glucose intolerance are exceptionally likely, and hence a fat source must be available. When using 5% dextrose infusions, this will only provide <25% of the RER when administered at maintenance fluid rates.[1]

Parenteral nutrition administration
Aseptic placement of a dedicated catheter is required in order to administer PN. When placing a cath-

eter for TPN, a central venous (jugular) catheter is required. The use of multi-lumen catheters is advocated, as they can also be used for blood sampling and the administration of fluids and intravenous medications, as a separate lumen is required for each purpose. As with enteral assisted feeding methods, TPN should be instituted gradually over a 3-day period. Flow rates of other fluids being concurrently administered should be adjusted accordingly.

Once the animal is consuming adequate nutrient intake voluntarily, the PN can be discontinued. TPN needs to be discontinued gradually over a 6- to 12-hour period. PPN can be discontinued abruptly. All animals receiving TPN or PPN should be closely monitored. Daily weighing of the animal must occur, with monitoring of temperature, pulse and respiration throughout the day. The catheter site should also be monitored, and handled aseptically.

Key points

- Assess bodyweight on a daily basis.
- Always consider the use of assisted feeding methods.

CASE STUDY 8.1

A 6-month-old Jack Russell terrier puppy was admitted as an emergency case after falling into a bath of scalding water. The puppy was initially treated with emergency first aid medical care, of intravenous fluid therapies, antibiotics and analgesia, and first aid treatment for the scalds. The interior of the puppy's mouth was severely scalded (Fig. 8.11) and voluntary consumption of food was impossible. In this case it was necessary to first investigate the degree of scalding that the puppy's mouth and throat had undergone, in order to decide which form of supportive feeding could be instigated. Through endoscopy it was visualized that the pharyngeal and cranial oesophagus had undergone some scalding, and a PEG tube was therefore placed. Scalds have an illness factor the same as for burns (1.5–2.0 × RER), and therefore a high-energy recovery diet was used.

CASE STUDY 8.2

A 4-year-old English springer spaniel was presented to the practice with a stick injury to the mouth. The referring practice had attempted to remove any stick fragments, but some were remaining, causing a localized infection to the back of the mouth. Further surgery in an attempt to remove the wood fragments was unsuccessful. The dog was administered broad-spectrum antibiotics, but soon deteriorated. The infection had spread and the dog was now anorexic. It was placed on intravenous fluid therapy, and decisions were being made on how to commence nutritional support. Within 24 hours the dorsal surface of the dog's neck had sloughed (Fig. 8.12). This removed the ability to use TPN because it was not possible to achieve access to a central vein. Enteral feeding methods were not used because the infection involved the digestive system. PPN was initiated instead, through the cephalic vein. An illness factor of 3 was used due to the severity of the sloughing. High levels of proteins were being lost. High levels of analgesia and anti-microbials were used in this case. The animal was euthanized on humane grounds.

This unfortunate case highlights the decisions that have to be undertaken when choosing a method of nutritional support. The RER is determined by the illness factor, which is as individual as the animal. Readjustments to the calculations need to occur, to ensure good health and recovery.

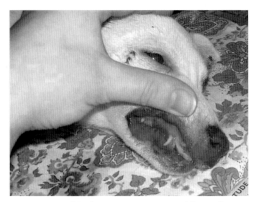

Figure 8.11   Scalded puppy: severe scalds to the nose and mucous membranes.

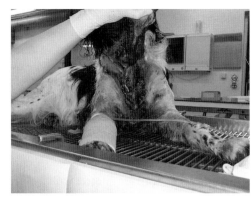

Figure 8.12   A stick injury has caused massive sloughing, causing difficulties for placement of nutritional support.

References

1. Chan D. Parenteral nutritional support. In: Ettinger SJ, Feldman EC, eds. Textbook of veterinary internal medicine. Volume 1. 6th edn. Dt Louis, Missouri: Elsevier Saunders; 2005:586–591.

2. Geor RJ. Nutritional support of the sick adult horse. In: Pagan JD, Geor RJ, eds. Advances in equine nutrition II. Kentucky: Kentucky Equine Research; 2001:429–452.

3. Buffington CAT, Holloway C, Abood SK. Manual of veterinary dietetics. Missouri: Elsevier Saunders; 2004.

4. Agar S. Small animal nutrition. Edinburgh: Butterworth-Heinemann; 2003.

5. Harcourt-Brown F. Anorexia in rabbits 2: diagnosis and treatment. In Practice 2002; (Sept):450–467.

6. Harris PA, Frape DL, Jeffcott LB, et al. Equine nutrition and metabolic diseases. In: Higgins AJ, Wright IM, eds. The equine manual. London: Saunders; 1995:123–186.

7. Michel KE. Deciding who needs nutritional support. Waltham Focus 2006; 16(3):17–21.

8. Ditchburn L. The principles of PEG feeding in the community. Nursing Times 2006; 102(22):43–45.

9. Remillard RL, Armstrong PJ, Davenport DJ. Assisted feeding in hospitalised patients: enteral and parenteral nutrition. In: Hand MS, Thatcher CD, Remillard RL, et al., eds. Small animal clinical nutrition. 4th edn. Missouri: Mark Morris Institute; 2000:351–399.

10. Torrance AG. Intensive care – nutritional support. In: Kelly N, Wills J, eds. BSAVA manual of companion animal nutrition and feeding. Gloucester: BSAVA Publications; 1996:171–180.

9
Dental disease

Dogs and cats

The incidence of dental disease shows that it is the most common problem suffered by adult dogs and cats: 85% of dogs, and 70% of cats over the age of 3 suffer from some form of dental disease.[1] The development of periodontal disease is dependent on the host's immunity and inflammatory responses to plaque on the tooth's surface.[2]

The diet of the animal can play an important preventative and therapeutic role. The type of food consumed, its texture and composition directly affect the oral environment. The use of dental diets and their overall effectiveness depends on three factors.

1. The level of plaque present on the teeth, and the animal's response to the plaque on the teeth (gingivitis).

2. The owner's ability to accomplish dental homecare on the pet (e.g. tooth brushing).

3. The selection of the methods of oral homecare by the veterinary practice for the owner. Consideration should include products that are most likely to ensure compliance; this also includes cost of the products.

Dental diets are designed with a few different mechanisms. The kibble size is influential; large kibbles force the animal to chew the kibble, increasing chewing activity. The texture of the diet, as with those that are high in fibre, have been shown to be beneficial in the removal of plaque and calculus from the teeth (Fig. 9.1). Calculus is formed by the mineralization of plaque, in particular by calcium. Calcium is secreted in the saliva, and is thus part of the reason why certain teeth have larger calcium deposits than other teeth. These teeth tend

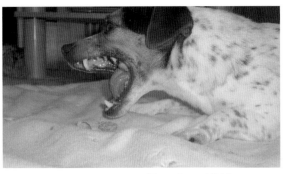

Figure 9.1 Demonstration of how large kibbles encourage chewing.

to be located next to salivary ducts. The use of polyphosphates in the diet is to bind the calcium from the saliva making it unavailable for the formation of calculus. The calcium is then released as normal in the digestive tract and absorbed by the animal. The use of polyphosphates is more effective when coating the kibble rather than incorporated into the kibble.[1]

The aims of dietary management of dental disease include:

- encouraging chewing – this can be achieved by using kibbles of different sizes
- limiting the components of plaque
- limiting mineralization of plaque to tartar (calculus)
- antimicrobial action.

Clinical nutrition
Carbohydrates
The use of fibre in the kibble is proven to reduce plaque and calculus accumulating on the tooth, but other forms of carbohydrates in high levels can be detrimental. The plaque bacteria utilize fermentable carbohydrates, like glucose, as a source of energy. Caries can form, because the by-products of this process are acidic and cause demineralization of the enamel.[3] Changes in the diet along with dental homecare can prevent the formation of caries in dogs. Caries in the cat has not been reported.[3]

Protein
A diet deficient in protein has been shown to cause degenerative changes in the periodontium. As protein deficiencies rarely occur in dogs and cats, this is not of practical consideration as a typical cause of periodontal disease. In some diets, protein levels are moderately reduced in order to limit the components of plaque.

Vitamins and minerals
Calcium and phosphorus consumed in unbalanced ratios can lead to secondary nutritional hyperparathyroidism, and significant loss of alveolar bone. The loss of bone can support the progression of periodontitis. Moderately reducing the levels of calcium in the diet, or its availability, can help limit the mineralization of plaque to tartar. The addition of polyphosphates (calcium chelating agents) can produce significant reduction in tartar formation ($\sim 45\%$).[4] Zinc has both antibacterial and healing properties (promotes a healthy epithelium).[5] Zinc salts can also inhibit the formation of tartar.

Vitamins C and A can also aid in dental problems, and are sometimes supplemented in dental diets. Vitamin C is important in the production collagen, which is the main protein found within the gums. Vitamin A aids in protecting the epithelium.

Feeding a dental diet
The use of diets is aimed primarily at preventing and removing small amounts of plaque and calculus. If the animal has larger amounts of calculus or periodontal disease, dental descaling and polishing will be required. Prophylactic diets, chews and tooth brushing can be recommended after dentistry. Most diets designed for dentistry are based around a senior lifestage diet, and those animals that require a diet with a high energy density may require additional calories from another source.

Dental hygiene chews are widely used, mainly due to the ease of compliance. Owners love the idea that they are giving their pet a treat, alongside it being a preventative treatment. Guidance does need to be followed with the use of these dental chews. Chews that are based on a rice flour formula are high in calories. Manufacturers' guidelines state that up to a third of the daily food ration needs to be removed if a chew is given. Rawhide-based chews have limited calorific value, but the chew should be removed when it becomes small enough for the dog to attempt to swallow it. Choking can easily occur at this stage, and supervision of the dog is recommended.

Rabbits

Diet of rabbits has been blamed for the cause of the majority of gastrointestinal and dental disorders. Problems such as myiasis (fly strike) can be attributed to the diarrhoea that the rabbit might have been suffering from. The dentition of rabbits is described in detail in earlier sections, and teeth are thought to grow at approximately 3 mm per week. Adequate levels of mastication are required in order to prevent overgrowth of the incisors and molars. Even a slight overgrowth of the incisors in rabbits can cause the alignment of the jaw to alter slightly. This can result in overgrowth of the molars with spur formation. Correction of the problem, via dentistry, will need to be performed, but the cause of the teeth overgrowth will also need to be addressed. Client education on the correct types of foods that rabbits should be fed is important. The use of coarse mixtures should be avoided, as selection of the highly palatable high-sugar pieces can occur, with a subsequent avoidance of the healthier high-fibre pieces. If concentrates are to be fed, pellets are recommended, and should only comprise a very small portion of the diet. The majority of the diet should be made up of hay, grasses and vegetables.

Clinical signs of dental disease in rabbits include:

- malocclusion causing overgrowth of the teeth, most notably the incisors
- salivation, commonly noted as a wet chin or dewlap
- poor body condition
- the appearance of hunger, but a disinclination or inability to eat
- asymmetrical or lumpy mandibles.

Owners should be encouraged to examine their rabbit's teeth on a weekly basis in order to identify any problems.

Creating a soft chewing environment for rabbits can be exceptionally beneficial. Providing objects such as cardboard, wood, dried pine cones, unlaquered wicker baskets and straw mats will aid in maintaining dental health.[6]

Equines

Equine dentition has evolved in order to consume a herbivorous diet. To create a continuous grinding occlusal surface, a narrowing of the interdental spaces has occurred. Ridges and troughs are also present on the occlusal surface running transversely in order to create an abrasive surface. These adaptations along with continuous eruption of the teeth have enabled the horse to maximize the efficacy of mastication.

Problems can arise when abnormal wear occurs, due to genetic make-up, trauma, age, incorrect diet or limited dental care. Poor condition, colic and malnutrition can develop when insufficient mastication occurs. Specific wear patterns can become apparent and include:

- *Wave mouth* – exaggerated development of the normal troughs and ridges of the occlusal surfaces.
- *Step mouth* – marked height variations in adjacent teeth.
- *Smooth mouth* – more commonly found in geriatric horses. Develops as teeth are lost or worn down to the gingival surface. This can also occur when the teeth have been over-rasped.
- *Anisognathism* – due to the differences of distance separating the dental arcades, which should be ~30%. Dental hooks can occur due to irregular wear. Regular (biannual) rasping is required in order to prevent occlusal dental problems of this nature.[7]

Periodontal disease usually occurs because of abnormal wear or abnormal dental eruption. Food material accumulates between individual teeth, causing pain and quidding. The gingival recess can become eroded and/or enlarged and can lead to food impactions. As the supporting alveolar bone becomes infected and eroded, and the periodontium becomes weaker, the abnormal shearing forces created during mastication can loosen teeth and accelerate any damage that is occurring.[7]

For any herbivore, regular dental examinations are required, along with any preventative care.

Nutrition is of the highest importance as normal wear of the teeth is required. Diets that necessitate the continuous grinding that the animal's teeth have adapted to through evolution are recommended. A high-fibre hay/grass based diet is ideal. In cases of diastema and smooth mouth, long fibre sources should be avoided in the diet.

Key points

Cats and dogs
- Encourage the animal to chew the diet.
- Avoid diets high in simple sugars (e.g. human foods, sweets).
- Initiate a daily oral hygiene plan.

Rabbits and horses
- Feed a diet that allows for the normal wear of the teeth.
- Advise on 6-monthly dental checks, including rasping/burring of the teeth if required.

CASE STUDY 9.1

A 5-year-old English bull terrier showed on annual vaccination to have a moderate level of plaque build-up on the teeth. This had started to cause gingivitis. The owner could not afford for the animal to undergo a dental procedure and general anaesthetic. The owner had previously failed with home dental care. A recommendation was given for a complete dental diet, which increases the necessity to chew the kibble (this dog tended to swallow dry kibbles whole) by having a large kibble size with fibre alignment to aid in plaque removal.

The owner fed the diet solely for a period of 8 weeks. When the dog was re-presented to the practice the quantity of tooth surface plaque had considerably reduced. This was shown to the owner with use of plaque-disclosing swabs. The dog's plaque-responsive gingivitis had also started to reduce.

References

1. Furniss G. The role of nutrition in the dental care of dogs and cats. Veterinary Review 2006; 11:450–454.
2. Tutt C. Tooth friendly diets. UK Vet 2006; 11(6):78–80.
3. Gorrel C, Derbyshire S. Veterinary dentistry for the nurse and technician. Edinburgh: Elsevier Butterworth-Heinemann; 2005.
4. Servet E, Hendriks W, Clarke D. Taking care of cats' teeth – kibbles can be useful in the prevention of periodontal disease. Waltham Focus 2003; 13(3):32–35.
5. Dethioux F, Marniquet P, Petit P, et al. How can we combat mouth disorders? Focus Special Edition: Preventative nutrition for major health risks in cats 2005; 29–36.
6. Harvey C. Oral health in rabbits. 2006 Online. Available: http://www.rabbit.org
7. Greet TRC, Howarth S. The ear, nose and throat. In: Higgins AJ, Wright IM, eds. The equine manual. London: Saunders; 1995:325–354.

10
Dermatological disease

The classification and diagnosis of nutritionally related skin disorders are initially based on a detailed dietary history and food evaluation. Dietary induced skin problems include food intolerances, primary and secondary nutrient deficiencies and nutrient toxicities.[1] The use of a diet history sheet can prove to be beneficial in obtaining all the necessary information. A full dietary history needs to include specific commercial foods, all snacks and treats, supplements, chewable/palatable medications and vitamins, chew toys, human foods and any food that the animal may have access to (Appendix 3). The use of a food diary can be helpful, as with obese animals.

The terms food allergy and food hypersensitivity should be reserved for those adverse reactions to food that have an immunological basis. Food intolerance refers to adverse food reactions due to non-immunological mechanisms. Dermatologists suggest that only 1–6% of all dermatoses seen in practice relate to adverse food reactions, and that food allergies constitute 10–20% of allergic responses in dogs and cats[1] (Fig. 10.1), confirming that a full dermatological work-up is required before a nutritional factor can be entirely confirmed. It is commonplace for owners to self-diagnose their pet's food allergy or intolerance, even before seeing the veterinary surgeon.

The skin is the largest organ of the body and has a heavy demand on bodily nutrient supply. When factors become suboptimal, it is usually the skin that becomes the first organ to demonstrate deterioration. The owner can easily detect signs of deterioration: loss of coat sheen; coat shedding; the coat can become greasy and scurf at the skin surface can be evident. Insufficiencies in the diet can

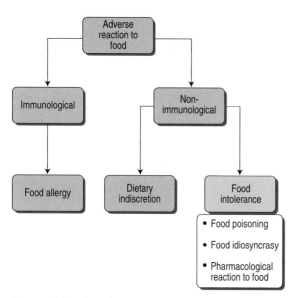

Figure 10.1   Flow diagram demonstrating different causes of adverse reactions to food.

be multifactorial and are displayed in Table 10.1. Allergic reactions to dietary constituents can result in hives. Hives can sometimes arise when 'rich' feeds are suddenly introduced into the diet.[2]

Aims of nutritional management include:

- help to avoid common food allergens
- using a highly digestible diet to help limit the amount of undigested protein passing through the gastrointestinal tract, which could provoke an allergic reaction.

Clinical nutrition

Fats

A common recommendation for atopic dermatitis is the supplementation of the diet with omega (n)-6 and omega (n)-3 essential fatty acids (EFA). Dietary supplementation has been shown to normalize

Table 10.1   Deficiencies and their effect on the skin in the dog[3]

Nutrient elements	Function in relation to the skin and coat	Minimum canine requirement (per MJ)	Clinical signs of insufficiency
Protein	Structure and pigment of keratinocytes and hair, component of sebum and sweat	9.6 g	Depigmentation of skin and hair, dry coat, hair loss
Lipids	Energy, precursors of eicosanoids, components of membrane phospholipids	3.3 g	Dull, dry coat, alopecia, greasy skin, pruritus
Linoleic acid	Maintenance of effective cutaneous barrier	0.66 g	Dry, scaly skin
Zinc	Metalloenzyme component, RNA and DNA polymerase co-factor	3.0 mg	Crusting/scaling of skin, erythema, alopecia
Copper	Melanin and keratinocyte synthesis	0.3 mg	Hypopigmentation and dry rough coat
Vitamin E	Antioxidant, stabilizer of cell membranes	1.8 IU	Scale, erythema, alopecia
Vitamin A	Cell growth and differentiation, keratinization process	245.5 IU	Hyperkeratinization, scaling, alopecia
Biotin	Metabolic enzyme co-factor	–	Facial alopecia and crusting
Riboflavin	Metabolic enzyme co-factor	0.15 mg	Dry, flaky dermatitis, swollen cracked lips
Niacin	Metabolic enzyme co-factor	0.72 mg	Pruritic dermatitis
Pyridoxine	Metabolic enzyme co-factor	0.07 mg	Dull, waxy coat and facial alopecia

the cutaneous fatty acid profile and improve the clinical signs in dogs with seborrhoea. EFA fulfil a number of roles in the body and skin. These include binding water into the stratum corneum, forming the epidermal permeability barrier, acting as antioxidants, and providing substrate for eicosanoids such as prostaglandin and leukotrienes. n-3 fatty acids compete with those of the n-6 series for the same enzymes, so n-3 supplementation will inhibit formation of arachidonic acid and its pro-inflammatory metabolites[4] (Fig. 10.2). The correct ratio of n-6 to n-3 fatty acids needs to be maintained within the diet. It is recommended that optimal levels be between 5:1 and 10:1 in the dog.[5] The understanding of dietary n-6:n-3 fatty acid ratios is less well defined in the cat and other species.[5] Fatty acid supplements commonly administered include starflower/borage, evening primrose and corn oils, which are high in levels of n-6 fatty acids. Cold-water marine fish, meat,

linseed and soya contain high levels of n-3 fatty acids. Dietary poly-unsaturated fatty acids (PUFA) have also been used in the management of certain inflammatory conditions, including allergic skin disease and arthritis.

Vitamins and minerals

Vitamin deficiencies are rarely diagnosed, and due to the large quantity of animals being fed a commercially balanced diet are unlikely. Any deficiencies are more likely to be a consequence of a genetic enzyme defect, or an absorption problem. Vitamin deficiencies may occur in animals receiving a fat-restricted diet or that have poor fat absorption. Some dietary components can also inactivate specific vitamins. For example, avidin in raw egg whites will bind biotin. Excessive amounts of the water-soluble vitamins can also be lost if the animal is suffering from polyuria. Vitamin A-responsive dermatosis is entirely confined to cocker spaniels, and is a rare condition. The condition is characterized by focal areas of follicular plugging with accumulation of keratin. Daily doses of 10 000 IU of vitamin A are required to resolve these lesions.[6]

Absolute dietary deficiencies of zinc are considered rare. More commonly there is a relative deficiency due to interaction or an inability to utilize the ingested zinc. Absorption can be inhibited by iron, copper and calcium, and reduced by intestinal phytate and inorganic phosphate. Calcium, iron and copper all compete with zinc absorption. Animals that receive high levels of calcium in their diet are those more likely to present with zinc deficiencies. These animals tend to be large or giant breeds that receive over-supplementation of calcium during growth periods. Specific breeds such as Siberian huskies and Alaskan malamutes appear to be unable to absorb adequate quantities of zinc. Bull terriers can suffer from lethal acrodermatitis, a metabolic inability to utilize zinc. This can result in systemic signs such as emaciation, stunting and immunocompromise. Zinc supplementation with oral zinc sulphate at 10 mg/kg BW, or zinc methionate at 1.7 mg/kg BW once daily with food is the treatment of choice for the breed.[5] Supplementation for other breeds may be required for the period until any dermatological lesions resolve, providing that the animal is placed on a nutritionally

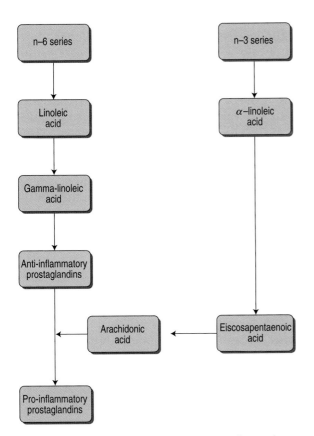

Figure 10.2 Inhibition of inflammatory pathways by supplementation of EPA.

balanced complete diet. Some may require lifelong supplementation.

Proteins

When designing or recommending an elimination diet, certain characteristics need to be taken into consideration. A limited number of protein sources are required, along with the protein from a novel source. Excessive levels of protein should be avoided; the protein present needs to be of a digestibility greater than 87%. Hydrolysed protein can be used, as digestibility is high. Digestibility is an important factor because free amino acids and small peptides make poor antigens. The diet needs to be free of additives and excessive levels of vasoactive amines, whilst still being nutritionally adequate for the animal's lifestage and body score.

Hydrolysed diets are advantageous as they remove the absolute necessity of finding the primary causal agent of the food allergen. Hydrolysed diets work by taking a protein and reducing it in size through hydrolysis. When the hydrolysed protein is then ingested, the body no longer recognizes the protein as an antigen, and the allergic immune response is not initiated.

Carbohydrates

The use of carbohydrates in the diet also needs to be limited. In many elimination diets a novel carbohydrate source is also used. Many carbohydrate sources used include rice, potato and tapioca.

Feeding an elimination food (dermatological and gastrointestinal disease)

The main diagnostic method for nutritional adverse food reactions is dietary elimination trials. Either a commercial product or a homemade diet can achieve the purpose of these trials. It must be noted that homemade diets are likely to be nutritionally inadequate for maintenance requirements. Most homemade diets lack a source of calcium, essential fatty acids, vitamins and other micronutrients. These diets also contain excessive levels of protein. If the owner is insistent on the use of a homemade diet, guidance on constructing a balanced diet is required from the veterinary practice.

In order to make a diagnosis of nutritional adverse food reactions, only the elimination food can be used. The trial needs to be performed for several weeks to months, and full dedication from the owner is required.

Elimination trials can prove to be extremely useful when diagnosing the causal nutritional agent in both dermatological and gastrointestinal disease. A strict elimination trial protocol does need to be adhered to, and the owner and anyone in contact with the animal needs to be aware of this. No other foodstuffs, other than the elimination food, should be ingested over this period. This includes treats, flavoured vitamins, chewable/palatable medications, fatty acids supplements and chew toys. Advice must be clearly conveyed to the owner when discussing the use of an elimination food trial. Many owners do not realize that when feeding a specific protein (e.g. lamb) and carbohydrate-sourced diet, the additional feeding of that specific protein (the lamb) in another form (e.g. processed) should not occur. The patient is fed the controlled diet for 4–12 weeks for dermatological disease. A shorter period of 2–4 weeks is usually satisfactory in gastrointestinal disease. The degree of clinical improvement during the elimination trial will be 100%, only if food sensitivity is the sole causal agent. These trials are often difficult to interpret in dermatological disease. This is due to concurrent allergic skin disease. These patients may only partially respond to an elimination trial. Confirmation of a diagnosis can be made of an adverse food reaction when the clinical signs reoccur within 10–14 days after the animal is challenged with its original diet.

Equine dermatology

Food allergy in the horse is rare, but should be considered as one of the differential diagnoses for horses presenting with chronic urticaria and/or pruritus.[7] It is commonly held that high-protein diets may lead to the development of cutaneous papules, often referred to as feed bumps, sweet feed bumps or protein bumps. The concept of the level of protein in the diet, rather than the presence of a certain type, does evoke scepticism in the light of knowledge of allergies in other species. However, reducing the plane of nutrition can appear to result in resolution of lesions in some animals.[8]

Diagnosis is based on feeding an elimination diet, as in small animals. Three to four weeks is a suggested period of time for the duration of the trial. Improvement on the restricted diet is not sufficient to make the diagnosis of a food allergy. Dietary challenge and provocation are required in order for confirmation.

Key points

- Always rule out any other differential diagnosis before initiating elimination food trials.
- Take a complete and honest dietary history.
- When using an elimination diet it must be adhered to 100% or its use is severely limited in order to make a solid diagnosis.
- In order to confirm dietary intolerance, a challenge in the food trial must have been used.

CASE STUDY 10.1

A 7-year-old domestic shorthaired cat was referred with severe pruritus and self-trauma. The cat's case had been previously worked up by the referring vet, and obvious causes such as flea allergic dermatitis (FAD) had been eliminated. The referral vet worked up the case thoroughly and ruled out any diagnosis of exoparasite, dermatophytosis or allergy to any exoparasite. The cat was placed on an elimination food trial, which involved the use of a novel protein and energy source, in this case venison and pea. Over a 3-month period the cat's health dramatically improved; there was, however, a relapse that resolved itself within a couple of weeks. The cause of this relapse was never found, but was thought to be due to the cat eating some of the neighbour's cat's diet. Once the cat had recovered from this relapse, a challenge was made to the diet, and the cat again showed the initial clinical symptoms, thus confirming a food allergy.

References

1. Roudebush P, Guilford WG, Shanley KJ. Adverse reactions to food 4. In: Hand MS, Thatcher CD, Remillard RL, et al., eds. Small animal clinical nutrition. 4th edn. Missouri: Mark Morris Institute; 2000:431–454.
2. Frape DF. Equine nutrition and feeding. 2nd edn. Oxford: Blackwell Science; 1998.
4. Lloyd DH. Nutrition and the skin. Dermatology for veterinary nurses. 17th ESVD-ECVD Congress Veterinary Dermatology. Copenhagen: 2001: 145–153.
5. Coatesworth J. Essential fatty acids and canine atopy. UK Vet Companion Animal 2006:63–64.
6. Davenport GM, Reinhart GA. Overview: the impact of nutrition on skin and hair coat. Recent advances in canine and feline nutrition. Volume III. Iams Nutrition Symposium Proceedings 2000:3–21.
7. Harvey RG. Nutrition and skin disorders. In: Kelly N, Wills J, eds. BSAVA manual of companion animal nutrition and feeding. Gloucester: BSAVA Publications; 1996:153–160.
8. Littlewood JD. Food allergy and urticaria: fact or fiction? Proceedings of the BEVA Specialist Days on Behaviour and Nutrition. September 1999:73–77.
9. Logas DB, Barbet JL. Diseases characterised by wheals, papules or small nodules. In: Colohan PT, Merritt AM, Moore JN, et al., eds. Equine medicine and surgery. 5th edn. St Louis: Mosby; 1999:1868–1946.

11
Endocrine disorders

DIABETES

Diabetes mellitus is a complex disease, with stabilization of blood glucose levels being affected by the confounding disease processes, efficacy of the primary disease control treatment, diet and exercise programme and weight control. Thus a full history of the animal including all these factors must be taken. There are several possible causes of diabetes mellitus, including pancreatitis, obesity, drugs (glucocorticoids, progestins), concurrent illness (hyperadrenocorticism, acromegaly), genetics, immune-mediated insulitis, infections and islet amyloidosis. Obtaining an ideal body condition score (BCS) in both cats and dogs is required. Obesity increases the risk of non-insulin-dependent diabetes mellitus (NIDDM) in cats by fourfold. Obese diabetic animals may have difficulty losing weight. Stabilization of the diabetes is the initial aim, followed by a conservative weight loss programme.

Underweight animals once stabilized should be fed a modest increase in calories in order to promote repletion. Dietary therapy can only improve glycaemic control, but emphasis should be placed on adjustment of the insulin (or oral hypoglycaemic) dosage and schedule, and control of concurrent disease.[1]

A scheme in order to classify diabetes mellitus in human medicine has been proposed,[2] and in many texts this has been translated to the veterinary medical field:

1. Insulin-dependent diabetes mellitus (IDDM or type 1)

2. Non-insulin-dependent diabetes mellitus (NIDDM or type 2)

3. Secondary diabetes mellitus (type S), as in concurrent diseases

4. Gestational diabetes

5. Impaired glucose tolerance

6. Previous abnormality of glucose tolerance (type PrevAGT).

Dietary manipulation of IDDM and NIDDM (type 1 and 2 respectively) will be discussed in this chapter.

With IDDM the beta cells within the pancreas lose their ability to secrete insulin. This can be congenital or as a result of pancreatitis or prolonged disease of the pancreas. Exogenous insulin administration is required as the treatment. NIDDM is when insulin resistance occurs at the site of the peripheral tissues. Dysfunction of the beta cells can also be a causal factor of NIDDM (Fig. 11.1). The quantity of insulin secreted by the beta cells can be increased, decreased, or remain normal. In some texts, type 2 diabetes that resolves is classed as transient type 2 NIDDM. This is more commonly noted in obese cats when insulin resistance becomes established. Once the cat obtains and then maintains an ideal body condition score, NIDDM can resolve itself. If the beta cells also become exhausted, a period of exogenous insulin administration may be required. The beta cells can start secreting insulin after a period of time. Hyperglycaemia is toxic to beta cells and aggravates the situation by further reducing insulin secretion. This mechanism can also explain why the more obese the animal and the longer that this animal has been obese the greater the incidence of the onset of diabetes. There are many factors that can predispose the animal to insulin resistance, and these are detailed in Box 11.1.

Nutritional aims are to:

■ aid in the reduction of postprandial hyperglycaemic spikes

■ maintain optimal BCS and hydration levels

■ supply the required amounts of nutrients and calories for the specific lifestage, including those lost through clinical symptoms (e.g. the water-soluble vitamins if polyuria is present).

Clinical nutrition

Water

A clinical symptom of diabetes mellitus is polydipsia and polyuria. Obligatory losses of electrolytes, such as sodium, potassium, chloride, calcium and phosphorus, and the water-soluble vitamins will occur. Access to fresh water at all times is required, and in severe cases administration of parenteral fluid may be required. Monitoring fluid intake, if possible, is a good indicator of glucose control.

Box 11.1   Factors that can predispose to insulin resistance
■ Obesity
■ Hyperadrenocorticism (HAC/Cushing's)
■ Dioestrus
■ Diabetogenic medications
■ Acromegaly
■ Infections (e.g. dental or urinary)
■ Hyper- and hypothyroidism
■ Chronic renal failure
■ Congestive hepatic failure
■ Congestive cardiac failure
■ Hyperlipidaemia
■ Hypercalcaemia
■ Pancreatitis
■ Neoplasm

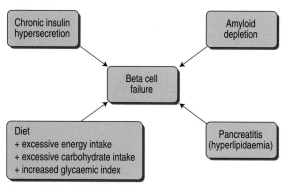

Figure 11.1   Physiopathology of insulin-resistant diabetes.

Proteins

Protein levels may need to be increased for diabetic dogs, especially in the quality of the proteins provided. This is due to losses of amino acids in the urine, a consequence of renal glomerulopathy or changes in hormonal signals. Excess protein levels need to be avoided, as renal damage can be enhanced.

Carbohydrates

Consumption of soluble or simple carbohydrates is the primary cause of rapid postprandial hyperglycaemic spikes. Diets need to avoid high levels of soluble carbohydrates, and the feeding of treats high in soluble carbohydrates should be stopped. Use of insoluble carbohydrates, fibre, has a positive effect on glycaemic control in dogs and cats. Diets that contain fibre, which has gelling properties, have an ability to slow the rate of presentation of nutrients (including glucose) to the body. This helps reduce the postprandial spike. The fermentation products of fibre, short-chain or volatile fatty acids, also modify the secretion of some of the digestive hormones and the sensitivity of tissues to insulin. Complex carbohydrates should provide ~50–60% of the calories in diets for cats and dogs.[1]

Felines are obligate carnivores and have a unique metabolism. Recent developments in feline nutrition for diabetic patients now recommend a reduced-carbohydrate diet. Initially, feeding a growth diet was the diet of choice, due to the relative protein increase and decrease in carbohydrate content. Specific diets aimed at diabetic cats have now been created. A decrease in carbohydrate content will also create an increase in percentage dry matter (DM%) fat content (Table 11.1). A high-protein, low-carbohydrate diet has been shown to enhance insulin sensitivity. Blood glucose levels should be monitored after dietary introduction as hypoglycaemia can result. This combination of high protein, low carbohydrate closely resembles the natural diet of a cat in the wild. In studies examining this dietary therapy it has been shown that insulin treatments could be discontinued in 15 out of 24 cats.[3]

Vitamins and minerals

Polyuria (a common clinical symptom of diabetes) will increase the loss of electrolytes and water-soluble vitamins. Magnesium and phosphorus are the most significantly lost. Chromium can be used to improve peripheral insulin sensitivity and glucose tolerance, though accurate studies on the use of chromium have not been conclusive. Vanadium, when dosed in pharmacological amounts, has insulin-like effects, though it causes gastrointestinal side effects, and chronic excessive intake may have toxic effects.

Feeding an insulin-dependent diabetic pet

On diagnosis of diabetes mellitus, dramatic changes to the animal's diet can be contraindicated. A high-carbohydrate diet should be avoided, as should semi-moist diets. These diets have a hyperglycaemic effect due to the increased levels of simple carbohydrates and other ingredients used as humectants (e.g. propylene glycol). Cost does play a deciding factor in choosing a diet for a diabetic patient, as does whether or not the animal eats the food. High-fibre diets are exceptionally useful in aiding stabilization of glucose control in dogs, but if the dog is unwilling to consume adequate amounts, this can be detrimental to the animal. An underweight

Table 11.1 Difference between a traditionally used high-fibre diet and a high-protein low-carbohydrate diet for feline diabetes sufferers

Diet	Carbohydrate		Protein		Fat		Fibre	
	DM(%)	g/100 kcal	DM(%)	g/100 kcal	DM(%)	g/100 kcal	DM(%)	g/100 kcal
Hills w/d	25	6.5	41	11	17	4.4	10.7	2.9
Hills m/d	15.7	3.9	52.8	13	19.4	4.8	6	1.5
Difference	62% ↓	60% ↓	24% ↑	15% ↑	13 ↑	9% ↑	56% ↓	51% ↓

DM, dry matter

animal will need a modified diet in order to gain weight, but this can only be achieved with insulin therapy. A high-fibre diet in these cases can also be detrimental.

Administration of exogenous insulin needs to be coordinated with times of feeding. Insulin regimens, whether insulin is being administered once or twice daily, will have a large effect on quantities being fed at each mealtime. If injected once daily, half the food should be fed at the time of injection, the remainder 8–10 hours later. Twice daily injections require meals containing half the daily calorific intake at the same time as insulin administration. The owner needs to be aware of the detrimental effects of feeding snacks and treats between meals. Milk should also be avoided due to the calorific intake. Timing of meals is not as critical in feline diabetic patients, and it is advised to continue feeding the cat in the way that it is used to (e.g. ad libitum). Cats that are fed set meals should receive one-third of the daily food requirement at the time of administration of the insulin. The remainder of the diet should be fed at the estimated peak action time of the insulin (when the glucose nadir occurs); this differs for each animal.

In cases of hypoglycaemia the owner can administer dextrose gels (Hypo-stop gel), or honey, jams or syrups to the mucous membranes of the mouth. This should only be recommended on advice from the veterinary surgeon once the owner has contacted the veterinary practice, or the blood glucose level has been measured. Use of an at-home glucometer can be exceptionally valuable, but obtaining sufficient blood for a test during a hypoglycaemic episode can be very difficult. This is due to a constriction of the peripheral blood supply, and in more severe cases shaking or convulsions. Depending on glycaemic control, smaller frequent meals may prove to be more beneficial in obtaining control. The use of mini-glucose curves in establishing nadir, length of insulin action and dietary effect is invaluable.

Feeding a non-insulin-dependent diabetic pet

Many animals that present with NIDDM are obese. A controlled weight-loss programme is required in these cases. Predisposition to hepatic lipidosis during rapid weight loss is of concern in cats. Once an ideal body condition score has been achieved in these animals, and glucose levels remain stable, it is important that they receive regular check-ups, including weighing. Use of a higher-fat and protein, decreased-carbohydrate diet has proved to be very useful in cats suffering from NIDDM.

The choice of diet will also depend on any secondary medical conditions. Renal dysfunction is commonly experienced when there has been a persistent hyperglycaemia. A low-salt diet would be a more preferable choice, but care should be taken as these diets have a higher carbohydrate content due to a restriction in protein levels.

Diabetes in horses and rabbits

Diabetes mellitus in horses and rabbits is considered rare. The most common form of diabetes in the horse is secondary diabetes, and has been reported following hyperadrenocorticism and in association with granulosa cell tumours. Recently the role of non-insulin-dependent diabetes has been identified as a potential problem in obese animals. Ponies with non-insulin-dependent diabetes will show improved insulin sensitivity on feeding a maintenance diet, especially in combination with an exercise programme.

Key points

- Establish the correct BCS.
- Establish insulin regimens prior to dietary changes.
- When establishing an insulin regimen only ever change one factor (e.g. food, insulin levels, timings, etc.) each time. These changes must be maintained for at least 1 week prior to a second change, as the body's physiological response takes time to fully adapt.
- Ensure plenty of fresh water is available at all times.

CASE STUDY 11.1

A 3-year-old entire bitch was presented with poly-dipsia (PD) and polyuria (PU). The dog was also polyphagic, and had chronic weight loss. Urinalysis showed marked glucosuria, and diabetes was confirmed with blood sampling. As the bitch was entire, an ovariohysterectomy was performed, as hormones released during oestrus can alter glucose metabolism. Postoperatively the bitch still displayed symptoms of diabetes, and insulin therapy was initiated. The dog's diet was adequate and stabilization on this diet was satisfactory. Once insulin therapy was started, clinical symptoms of PD/PU, polyphagia and glucosuria were all reduced. As the dog was underweight, BCS 2/5, slightly higher levels of diet were fed in order to aid the dog to reach its optimal weight.

Once the dog was stabilized and had reached its optimal weight and BCS, it was transferred to a higher-fibre diet. This would help to reduce the quantity of exogenous insulin that was being used. The dog made this transition very well, and the levels of insulin could be reduced by 2 IU, on each administration.

EQUINE METABOLIC SYNDROME

Equine metabolic syndrome (EMS) is characterized by obesity, insulin resistance and the increased risk of laminitis, and is a common endocrinopathic condition of mature horses.[4] The principal cornerstones of the therapeutic approach to EMS is through dietary management of obesity and exercise. The term EMS has been previously classified as 'hypothyroidism', 'syndrome X', peripheral Cushing's syndrome and pre-Cushing's syndrome.[5] The use of the term EMS is controversial and some prefer to use the term 'insulin resistance syndrome' in obese horses,[5] which can be compared to non-insulin-dependent diabetes. Unlike humans and cats, horses appear capable of sustaining high insulin output despite insulin resistance. Treatment of EMS includes reducing calorie intake, improving the lipid profile, improving glucose homeostasis (use of antidiabetic drugs) and lowering blood pressure.

The nutritional aims of the diet include:

- reduction of calorie intake that aids in weight loss
- helping to improve the lipid blood profile
- providing a diet that has a low glycaemic index.

Clinical nutrition

Carbohydrates

When feeding a horse with EMS, the most important aspect of dietary management is to limit the soluble carbohydrate content of the diet. The use of the glycaemic index (GI) can evaluate the level of soluble sugars within a certain foodstuff. The GI index is a tool used for describing the effect of a particular food on blood glucose concentration compared with a reference food. The reference food is usually glucose, which therefore has a GI of 100. Table 11.2 details the glycaemic index for certain foodstuffs. These data are extremely helpful, but can only be used as a guide when formulating the individual's diet. This is due to the huge variations in grass hay, depending on where it was grown, growing conditions, stage of growth when cut, and drying conditions. Each individual will also digest and metabolize foods differently. Some equine nutrition companies offer a simplified hay analysis, which identifies the sugar and NDF values of the hay.

Hay, which is low in non-structural carbohydrates (NSC) or simple sugars, should make up the majority

Table 11.2 Glycaemic index of commonly fed foods

Foodstuff	Glycaemic index
Glucose	100
Plain beet pulp	1
Rice bran	22
Bermuda hay	23
Alfalfa hay	26
Alfalfa cubes	30
Timothy hay	32
Wheat bran	37
Carrots	51
Vetch blend hay	53

of the diet. Other feeds such as carrots, apples, wheat bran, molasses added to beet pulp and fresh grass should be fed in restricted quantities to ensure the total diet is low in these sugars.[4] Soaking of the hay can also aid in reducing the NSC content, and the use of hot water has been found to be more beneficial than cold water. This is due to the solubility of the sugars in water being higher in warm water. If hard feeds do need to be fed in order to administer medications or supplements, the use of no-molasses/plain beet pulp should be recommended.

Fats

The addition of fats to the diet has been shown to decrease the glucose and insulin response in horses, though high-fat diets long term can worsen the effects of insulin resistance in ponies.[4] There are no current data supporting the use of fat/oil supplementation in the diet, and it should therefore be avoided. The use of monosaturated fats (e.g. olive oil) can be beneficial in controlling equine hypertriglyceridaemia.

Protein

High-protein diets should be avoided, as most amino acids can act as potent triggers of insulin release.[4] Adequate, but not excessive, protein levels are advisable; crude protein requirements are met when grass hay containing 7.5% protein is consumed at a rate of 2% BW/day. The essential amino acid lysine should be supplemented, as grass hays are often low in lysine.

Vitamins and minerals

Levels of vitamins and minerals need to reflect the particular lifestage and work level of the animal. Higher levels of specific nutrients could be beneficial in an antioxidant role.

References

1. Michel KE. Nutritional management of endocrine disease. In: Ettinger SJ, Feldman EC, eds. Textbook of veterinary internal medicine. Volume 1. 6th edn. St Louis, Missouri: Elsevier Saunders; 2005.
2. Stogdale L. Definition of diabetes mellitus. Cornell Vet 1986; 76:156–174.
3. Mazzaferro EM, Greco DS, Turner AS, et al. Treatment of feline diabetes mellitus using an α-glucosidase inhibitor and a low carbohydrate diet. J Feline Med Surg 2003; 5(3):183–189.
4. Johnson PJ. Are you feeding the wrong food or has your horse inherited the 'fat gene'? Dodson and Horrell 5th International Feeding Conference. Applied Session; 2005:5–18.
5. Johnson PJ. Equine metabolic syndrome: mechanisms of insulin resistance and the role of adipose tissue as an endocrine organ. Dodson and Horrell 5th International Feeding Conference. Scientific Session; 2005:29–41.

12
Gastrointestinal disorders

DOG, CAT AND RABBIT

The gastrointestinal tract (GIT) is a complex system; in chronic, acute or severe gastrointestinal (GI) disturbances diet can have a profound effect on GIT recovery and successful management of disease.[1,2]

Adverse reactions to food – GI

Food allergies (food hypersensitivity) have an immunological basis, and cause an adverse reaction to food or food additive. Food intolerances are non-immunological, where abnormal physiological responses to food or a food additive occur.[1] Specific food additives that are known to cause problems include onions and propylene glycol, which can cause haematological abnormalities in cats. Lactose intolerance is a relatively common metabolic adverse reaction in dogs and cats. Diarrhoea can develop when given cow's or even goat's milk, owing to the lactose content being higher than that of bitch's or queen's milk. Gluten sensitive enteropathy has been well documented in Irish setters.

The role of food allergies in canine and feline inflammatory bowel disease (IBD) is unknown. It is thought that hypersensitivity to food is involved in the pathogenesis of this syndrome. The use of elimination food trials often alleviates the signs of IBD, which does seem to imply that food allergies or food intolerances play a role in this syndrome.[1]

For further information on clinical nutrition for patients suffering from adverse food reactions, see Chapter 10.

Acute gastroenteritis and vomiting, or small bowel diarrhoea

Acute vomiting and diarrhoea are the most common reason why animals are presented to the veterinary practice. The definition of diarrhoea is an abnormal increase in frequency, water content or volume of faeces. This can result in the reduced absorption of nutrients, and the loss of water, electrolytes and water-soluble nutrients, which can lead to dehydration and acidosis. Acute diarrhoea can be subdivided into four different categories, which are described in detail in Table 12.1.

The cause of acute diarrhoea and vomiting is most commonly irritation of the gut mucosa by toxins and infections. The clinical symptoms of vomiting and diarrhoea are a response to remove the causal agent from the gastrointestinal tract. In some cases abrupt changes to the animal's diet can induce these symptoms. In these cases it is wise to stop feeding the new diet. Once the animal has returned to full health on the old diet, initiate a slow and correct transitional change. It is important to differentiate between small and large intestinal diarrhoea, as treatment can vary (Table 12.2).

Table 12.1 Classification and pathophysiology of diarrhoea[3]

Classification of acute diarrhoea	Pathophysiology	Common causes
Osmotic	Excess water-soluble molecules in the intestinal lumen result in osmotic retention of water. Diarrhoea occurs when the fluid volume overwhelms the absorptive capacity of the small intestine and colon	Sudden dietary change, malabsorption
Permeability (exudative)	Inflammation in the intestine can stimulate increased secretion of fluid and electrolytes, and impair absorption	Permeability can be affected by ulceration, especially in cases of neoplastic disease. Where severe damage is present serum protein and blood loss can also occur. Portal hypertension can also result in exudation of fluid into the intestinal lumen
Secretory	When the absorptive capacities of the small intestine and colon are exceeded. Resulting diarrhoea can be severe, and does not usually resolve with fasting	Toxin release by enteric infectious agents (e.g. *Giardia* spp., *Escherichia coli*)
Dysmotility	Diarrhoea can result in secondary alterations in motility, usually reduced intestinal motility	Ileus and abnormal dilation of the intestine can be physical, neuromuscular, metabolic or functional abnormalities, and can further promote diarrhoea as stasis allows for bacterial fermentation

Table 12.2 Differences between small and large intestinal diarrhoea in the cat and dog

Clinical symptom	Small intestinal diarrhoea	Large intestinal diarrhoea
Blood in faeces	Melaena	Heamatochezia
Frequency of defecation	Mild increase (< 3 × day)	Markedly increased (>3 × day)
Faecal volume	Large quantities	Small quantities
Faecal quality	Loose, watery, 'cow-pie'	Loose to semi-formed, 'jelly-like'
Urgency	Usually absent	Often present
Tenesmus	Rare	Common
Faecal mucus	Rare	Common
Dyschezia	Absent	May be present
Vomiting	May be present	May be present
Weight loss	Common	Rare
Flatus/borborygmi	May be present	May be present

Dietary management of cases of acute gastro-enteritis can initially include a period of starvation. (Also see Box 12.1 on 'Feeding through'.) A period of 24–48 hours can be given; this food deprivation allows the gastrointestinal tract to clear itself of the luminal contents, including the causal agents. It also aids in preventing mucosal cell abrasion, deprives opportunistic pathogenic bacteria of nutrients, prevents absorption of dietary antigens by a compromised mucosa, and may permit re-establishment of brush border enzymatic function. When starting the animal on a diet, a highly digestible diet should be fed using small frequent meals. This can be a home-made diet of lean chicken, or cottage cheese and rice. Specific veterinary diets do offer a more balanced nutritional meal, as they will cater for losses of electrolytes and vitamins through vomiting and diarrhoea. Electrolyte imbalances can quickly develop in animals with severe diarrhoea. Intravenous supplementation should also be provided when required, especially if the animal is vomiting.[3] Baby rice is an ideal carbohydrate source to use in these cases, but cats are less tolerant of carbohydrates and more tolerant of fats. An appropriate diet for this species would be of boiled chicken, or a specific veterinary diet.

Adsorbents are frequently used in these cases, and can be provided with the addition of pro- and prebiotics, and glutamine. The purpose of adsorbents is to bind bacteria and toxins, to protect the intestinal mucosa, and potentially for an

Box 12.1 Feeding through

In human medicine there is a continuing bank of evidence indicating that 'feeding through' diarrhoea with an appropriate diet can be beneficial. Comparisons can be difficult, as many cases of diarrhoea in man tend to be secretory, whereas osmotic diarrhoea is more common in dogs and cats.[4] The advantages of feeding through include maintaining mucosal health, reducing the risk of bacterial translocation, and aiding in the 'flushing out' of the causal factor. Feeding through should not be used in animals that are vomiting or severely dehydrated. The nutritional requirements of animals that are vomiting or have a non-functioning GIT should be met through parenteral nutrition. The obvious disadvantage is the risk of 'accidents' in the house, and the increase in faecal volume. Whether food is withheld or not, unlimited access to water must be maintained at all times. The use of oral rehydration solutions containing carbohydrates, peptides and electrolytes should be advocated in these cases. When using this method, feeding a diet that will not cause an inflammatory reaction in the future is important. Dietary antigens can cross the compromised gastrointestinal mucosa and set up a hypersensitivity reaction. Use of a novel protein and/or carbohydrate source should be recommended. Once the animal is well, and transferred to its original diet, it is unlikely to have any reactions to the original protein source.

antisecretory effect.[3] Kaolin has been traditionally used, but montmorillonite has been reported to be 20 times more effective than kaolin at absorbing pathogens.[3]

Anal glands and impactions

Anal gland impactions can occur when the dog or cat's diet is low or restricted in fibre. The inclusion of fibre in the diet provides a bulking agent, and allows a constant pressure on the glands at defecation, thus decreasing the risk of the glands becoming full. Glands that become over-full have a higher risk of becoming infected and/or impacted. Dietary management of these cases is necessary, and the inclusion of fibre in the diet is warranted. This can be achieved by feeding a higher-fibre diet, or by the addition of fibre-containing pellets.

Where anal gland surgery has been performed, the use of a low-residue (low-fibre) diet is advocated, in order to remove pressure from suture lines.

Borborygmus and flatulence

Borborygmus and flatulence are a very common occurrence in many dogs. This can be due to the diet, or the rapid consumption of the diet, which leads to aerophagia. Diets that are low-quality and poorly digestible can be problematic. Dietary change can be recommended in these cases. For dogs which consume their diet too quickly, the diet can be spread out on a flat surface, fed little and often, or have added water, all of which can aid in increasing consumption time.

Dietary management is concerned with decreasing the intestinal gas production by bacterial fermentation of undigested foods. Commercial products are available for reducing flatulence. These products can contain α-galactosidase, and reduce flatulence by improving digestion of non-absorbable carbohydrates.[5] Diets high in protein have also been implicated in increased levels of flatulence, as have vitamin and mineral supplements due to the increased intestinal microbial activity.[5] Veterinary medicines to counteract flatulence can contain antacids, aluminium hydroxide and magnesium trisilicate, as well as copper complexes of chlorophyllins. Clinical trials have clearly demonstrated efficacy in reducing wind and smells and relieving indigestion and gastric upset in the dog. The local antacid effect in the stomach promotes coalescence and removal of trapped gasses from the gut contents, thereby limiting their passage through into the later stages of the gastrointestinal tract.

Chronic diarrhoea

Chronic diarrhoea can be a clinical sign of a vast number of different problems. It is essential to determine the underlying cause so that specific treatments for each individual case can be initiated. Dietary management plays an important role in long-term management of these cases, as relapses can be frequent. As each case is different there is no one specific diet aimed at animals suffering from chronic diarrhoea. Recommendations of low-fat, single (novel) protein diets are given. Yet in some cases, a diet with a high fibre content is the diet of choice in resolving the clinical symptoms. The chronic diarrhoeal disorders such as inflammatory bowel disease (IBD), protein-losing enteropathy (PLE), antibiotic-responsive diarrhoea (ARD) and irritable bowel syndrome (IBS) will be discussed separately because of their significance in veterinary medicine.

Inflammatory bowel disease (IBD)
The management of IBD involves the combined use of anti-inflammatory medication alongside the use of a single novel protein diet. A full dietary history is required in order to ascertain what protein sources the animal has been exposed to in the past. Diets that contain novel protein sources such as venison or duck have proved to be beneficial, because lamb, which was initially used as a novel protein source, is now included in many lifestage diets that are marketed for animals with sensitive stomachs. When using an elimination diet, it is important to challenge the system to see if the original diet was the initial cause. See Chapter 10, 'Feeding an elimination food', for further details.

The use of fermentable fibre in these cases should not be underestimated. Colonic bacteria easily digest fermentable fibres, which in turn produce butyrate, a short-chain fatty acid (SCFA). Butyrate is the primary energy source for colonocytes, and thus helps to maintain gut health. Other SCFAs are also produced, which reduce the colonic pH, and thus reduce the risk of pathogenic bacteria colonizing the area. As the body absorbs the SCFAs there is an increase in the absorption of electrolytes and water from the colon.

When feeding an animal with IBD the nutritional goal is to provide adequate nutrient intake in order to meet the requirements of the individual, but also to compensate for ongoing losses through the gastrointestinal tract.

Protein-losing enteropathy (PLE) and lymphangiectasia

Lymphangiectasia is characterized by abnormalities of the intestinal lymphatic system. The condition can be as a primary defect of the lymphatic system, or secondary as a consequence of severe intestinal infiltrative disease (e.g. IBD, lymphosarcoma).[6] Lymphangiectasia is the most common cause of PLE in dogs and cats. Not all animals present with the clinical symptom of diarrhoea, but often present with progressive weight loss even with a good calorific consumption. The leaky intestinal lymphatics result in hypoalbuminaemia and loss of colloidal oncotic pressure.

When feeding animals with PLE the key is to control dietary fat levels. Long-chain triglycerides provide a major stimulus for intestinal lymph flow; the protein content of the lymph tends to increase with the dietary fat content. Limiting dietary fat content will reduce the lymphatic flow, reduce lacteal and lymphatic distension and thus minimize protein losses.[6] Dietary fat levels of < 10% dry matter base (DMB) for dogs and < 15% DMB for cats are recommended.[6] The protein levels of the diet are important; feeding a high-protein diet has been shown to be unsuccessful. The cause of the PLE is important, as in cases where severe IBD is the underlying cause, and care should be given when selecting a protein source. Protein should be of a high biological value, and levels in excess of 25% DMB for dogs and in excess of 35% DMB in cats have been recommended.[6]

Antibiotic-responsive diarrhoea (ARD)

ARD should be best managed with a combination of antibiotics and diet. The response to antibiotics will dictate the length of the course required. The antibiotic of choice in cases of ARD is tylosin or oxytetracycline.[7] Little research has been

conducted on the casual factors of ARD, yet speculation can be made that gastrointestinal factors must promote bacterial colonies that are causal agents for the diarrhoea. The use of prebiotics has been recommended in these cases in order to promote gastrointestinal health. Dietary manipulation should be considered if the animal is on an inappropriate diet that encourages growth of pathogenic bacteria.

Irritable bowel syndrome (IBS)

IBS is a difficult disorder to diagnose, and the diagnosis can be made only on elimination of all other causes of chronic diarrhoea. Clinical signs of IBS include bouts of abdominal pain and chronic large intestinal diarrhoea. The clinical signs can be intermittent, with stress also being a probable trigger factor. The addition of fibre to the diet has proven to be of a slight benefit in some cases.[8]

Colitis

Colitis is the most common cause of diarrhoea in the dog and cat. Colitis (inflammation of the colon) is characterized by the presence of mucus covering the faeces, and/or fresh blood. There are many causes of colitis, including stress. Many dogs have colitis diarrhoea when being hospitalized at veterinary practices, due to stress levels. Dietary management of mild cases is recommended, though in chronic or severe cases medical treatment may be required alongside dietary management. Modifications to the diet include:

- High-fibre diets that normalize the transit time and bind faecal water. Fibre also acts as a prebiotic, aiding the strains and populations of gut bacteria.
- Low-fibre, highly digestible diets that will aid in reducing the quantity of undigested food entering the colon.
- Hypoallergenic diets that can also be used when an intolerance or hypersensitivity is present.

When the initiating cause of the colitis is unknown, dietary modifications can be very much trial and error, as the first two (high fibre and low fibre) contraindicate each other. This should be relayed to owners so that they have a better understanding of the problem, and do not get frustrated with dietary managements. It is also recommended to advise owners that colitis is normally seen spasmodically, with intervals of normality between bouts.

Constipation/megacolon

Constipation in animals can be a clinical symptom of systemic disease, a response to nutrition or nutritional changes, or a consequence of damage to the pelvis. Constipation is characterized by absence, infrequency, or difficulty in defecation associated with retention of faeces within the colon and rectum.[5] The treatment and preventative management of constipation differ. The addition of fibre to the diet whilst the animal is constipated can compound the initial problem. Treatments can include enemas and laxatives. In order to prevent the reoccurrence of constipation a full history is required in order to identify the causal factor or factors. The water and fibre consumption of the animal needs to be ascertained. Maintenance of normal hydration levels is required; intake of water should be 40–60 ml/kg bodyweight per day. Recommendations to increase water intake in animals are detailed in Appendix 4. Fibre intake can be estimated from analysis of the pet food label.

Increasing the fibre content of the diet can improve constipation dramatically. Increasing the amounts of fibre in the diet can aid in increasing the water content of the faeces, intestinal transition rates and colonic motility. When increasing the fibre content of the diet, it should be remembered that fermentable and non-fermentable fibres should be included. The palatability of high-fibre foods can be decreased, and the transition to a fibre-enhanced veterinary therapeutic diet can be difficult. In some cases, remaining on the original diet and adding a fibre source can be utilized. Some animals can suffer side effects when changed to a high-fibre diet, if the transition is done too quickly. Flatulence and abdominal cramping are common side effects of the addition of the fermentable fibres. Some animals can develop megacolon or constipation when fed a diet with a moderate to high fibre content (>15% DM crude fibre). The transition to these diets should be made in increments of increasing fibre content. If such side effects do occur, then it is recommended that the fibre content be decreased by 5% DMB and the animal reassessed. Up to 10% fibre can be added to the diet without compromising its overall nutrient balance. Titration of the dietary fibre content of the diet can be achieved by the use of food combinations with diets of varying crude fibre content.

In situations of severe constipation or megacolon where colonic motility is not present, the use of a high-fibre diets is not recommended. In these cases a highly digestible diet (dry matter digestibility >90%) is the diet of choice. This will have an exceptionally low residue, whilst still providing adequate calories. In these cases the faecal production is minimal enough that removal of the faeces can be achieved via enemas once or twice weekly.

The use of medical therapies in the aid of constipation is an important adjunct to dietary management, and is suitable for mild to moderate constipation. Laxatives, lactulose, sorbitol and polyethylene glycol are poorly absorbed carbohydrates and prove to be very useful. These sugars are hydrolysed to fatty acids by the microflora of the colon, where they exert osmotic pressure and draw fluid into the colonic lumen. Colonic motility modifiers such as cisapride are also of use, especially in rabbits, the dose rate being 0.25 mg/kg BW, three to four times a day in dogs and cats.[1] Treatment of constipation and megacolon in animals is very much case specific, and can be dependent on the initiating cause.

Gastric dilation/volvulus

Gastric dilation/volvulus (GDV), or bloat, is thought to be the final common pathway of a variety of problems in certain predisposed breeds of large-breed dogs.[1] Gastric dilation is defined as the distension of the stomach with a mixture of air, food and fluid. GDV occurs when rotation of the stomach on its mesenteric axis happens. This entraps the gastric contents, whilst also compromising the vascular supply to the stomach, spleen and pancreas. Breeds which are predisposed are large-breed, deep-chested dogs, including Irish setters, Great Danes, standard poodles, Doberman pinschers, German shepherds and Saint Bernards. A body condition score (BCS) of ≤2/5 is also considered a risk factor for GDV. Males are twice as likely as females to develop GDV, and having a relative, especially a parent, that has experienced GDV greatly increases the risk. This can be as high as a 63% greater risk if a first-degree relative has suffered from GDV.[8]

Diet can play some role in susceptible animals, but no diet-related cause has been clearly identified.[1] Several dietary risk factors have been identified, and these include:

- Feeding only one meal per day.
- Postprandial exercise, especially vigorous exercise. Recommendations include avoiding exercise 1 hour before and 2 hours after a meal. Gentle exercise has been shown to improve gastrointestinal functioning, but must be restricted.
- Rapid consumption of food, leading to aerophagia. Rate of consumption can be reduced by placing the food on a flat baking tray, or spreading the dry food out on the floor.
- Food particle/kibble diameter of less than 30 mm.
- Consumption of large volumes of water. There needs to be limited availability of water immediately after feeding, if large consumptions do occur (more than one volume of water per volume of dry food). Mixing water with the dry diet in equal proportions can aid in preventing large volumes of consumption.
- Episodes of overeating.
- Dietary transitions that occur too quickly. All dietary transitions should be performed slowly; see Appendix 2 for details.

The consumption of dry diets has been blamed in the past for being a predisposing factor for GDV, but epidemiological studies have shown this to be an incorrect assumption.[6] Other dogs that seem to be predisposed to GDV are those which tend to be nervous and stressful. These dogs should always be fed alone, and in a quiet environment.

Feeding a dog predisposed to GDV

As there are no specific nutritional factors that have been established for gastric dilation (GD) or GDV, it is difficult to advise on a specific dietary regimen for these animals. The diet fed needs to provide all the adequate nutrients and energy requirements for that particular lifestage. The use of a highly digestible lower-fat diet has been advocated in these situations, as it is less fermentable and will have a shorter transit time through the stomach.

The daily management of the dog is important. This includes dividing the diet into small frequent meals, feeding from a raised level, avoiding exercise around the times of feeding, decreasing competitive feeding, feeding a mixture of moist and dry diets, increasing the time it takes for the dog to consume the diet and avoiding excess water consumption postprandially.

Owners should always be advised of the symptoms of GD or GDV in all breeds that are predisposed. In veterinary practices it is advisable to inform clients of this when they initially present their puppies at puppy clinics or at the initial vaccinations.

Hairballs in cats and rabbits

Hairballs are a common occurrence in cats, though cats with longer, thicker coats or those with fastidious grooming behaviour do tend to suffer more. Hairballs do not usually cause clinical disease, though vomiting can be a nuisance or even distressing for owners (Fig. 12.1). Laxatives and lubricants can be utilized, either with or without specialized diets, for the routine management of hairballs. The use of lubricants and laxatives should be limited, due to the interference with normal digestion and absorption of nutrients.

Hairballs are loose accumulations of hair and mucus which form in the digestive tract. In some cases the hair and mucus can combine with other

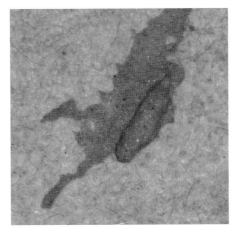

Figure 12.1 Vomited hairball from cat.

materials to form trichobezoars, which are much harder. Trichobezoars form within the stomach or intestines, and are less common in cats but are a common cause of anorexia in rabbits. If the trichobezoars become large enough, obstruction of the pyloric sphincter or intestines can occur. Hairballs are a common finding in rabbits due to their inability to vomit, and should be considered even in short-haired animals that present with anorexia. Often on palpation of the stomach a large doughy mass can be felt. Treatment for trichobezoars is based on breaking down the proteinaceous matrix that binds them together. Large trichobezoars must be removed via surgery or endoscopy.[1] If left, obstructions and ileus can occur. Survival after surgery of the digestive tract, particularly gastrotomy, is reportedly low in rabbits.[9] Hairballs in rabbits can be prevented by feeding a diet with adequate dietary fibre (>14% DM crude fibre), minimizing stress and boredom, and grooming the animal frequently.[8]

A common treatment for hairballs is pineapple juice and papaya juice, the supposed active ingredient being the enzyme bromelain (in pineapple juice) and papain (in papaya juice). There is no evidence to support this, and in truth the enzymes bromelain and papain are incapable of dissolving keratin, the main protein component of hair.[9,10] Simple sugars in the fruit juices may actually promote overgrowth of *Clostridium* spp.[10]

Ileus in rabbits

Adynamic or paralytic ileus (bowel dilation or intestinal stasis) can occur due to an impaired motor function, or secondary to an obstruction. Innervation can become defective due to a primary (rare) or a secondary cause. Secondary causes include gastroenteritis, trauma, stress, toxaemia or peritonitis. Ileus is often triggered by stress, with failure to recognize ileus and to provide immediate and appropriate treatment of the initial signs resulting in a 'downward spiral' in which each clinical sign generates another, more serious one (Figs 12.2 and 12.3). Ileus frequently presents as a clinical sign of many enteric diseases in the rabbit, with treatment of the clinical signs being the mainstay for rabbit enteric diseases.

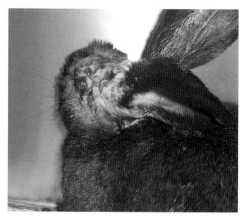

Figure 12.2   Stressful situations, in this case a pasteurella infection, can cause a reduction of GIT motility.

The treatment of enteric diseases is dependent on the clinical signs that are being presented. Body temperature needs to be obtained and heat pads or lamps used if required. The use of probiotics in the rabbit is now commonplace in cases of ileus, and even in postoperative cases where stress levels in the rabbit can induce complications. The use of *Lactobacillus* spp. in powders can be beneficial, but it should be noted that this species of bacterium is not part of the normal intestinal flora. It is, however, very efficient at competing with pathogenic bacteria for mucosal attachment when pH changes occur.[11] The most efficient way to re-establish the caecum with correct levels of flora is to use caecotrophs. This can be achieved by force-feeding a slurry of the caecotrophs via syringe or mixed with a herbivore recovery diet. The use of baby foods is not recommended as simple sugar levels can be too high in fruit-based foods. Vegetable baby foods can contain onion powders, which have been shown to cause haemolytic anaemia in some species. The use of exercise and gentle abdominal massage can be invaluable at reducing the signs of colic and can help stimulate peristalsis (Fig. 12.4).

Carbohydrates inhibit the release of motilin, a protein that helps regulate upper GI motility in rabbits by stimulating contractions of the small intestine. The administration of diets and products, which are high in simple sugars and digestible carbohydrates, may interfere with restoration of normal GI motility.[12]

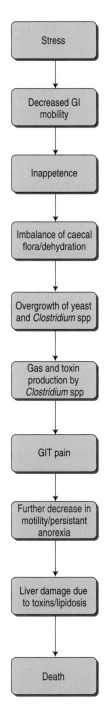

Stress

↓

Decreased GI mobility

↓

Inappetence

↓

Imbalance of caecal flora/dehydration

↓

Overgrowth of yeast and *Clostridium* spp

↓

Gas and toxin production by *Clostridium* spp

↓

GIT pain

↓

Further decrease in motility/persistant anorexia

↓

Liver damage due to toxins/lipidosis

↓

Death

Figure 12.3 Downward cascade of factors relating to ileus.[10]

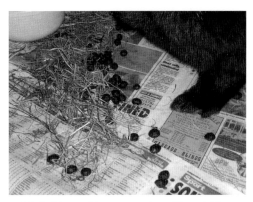

Figure 12.4 Normal faeces produced by rabbit.

The prevention of enteric problems in rabbits is ultimately the goal. Remember that ileus is not an illness, it is a symptom of an underlying disorder that has caused the rabbit enough stress or pain to caused hypomotility of the GIT. This revolves around the use of a high-fibre diet that mirrors what the rabbit would consume in the wild. Active encouragement to get the rabbit to eat is a vital part of nursing these animals. If the rabbit refuses to eat grass or hay, the use of fragrant fresh herbs can be beneficial. These include mint, basil, dill, tarragon, sage, fennel and parsley. In some cases getting the rabbit to take one bite of the offered food is all that is required to initiate self-feeding. This can be achieved by gently inserting a stem of grass or herb into the corner of the mouth, or even patting the piece of grass or herb on the rabbit's face until it gets annoyed and grabs the offending article.

Pharyngeal and oesophageal disorders

Animals with disease or disorders of the oesophagus are relatively uncommon, but can be profoundly debilitated due to malnutrition. Pharyngeal and oesophageal disorders can be divided into three different categories:

1. Mobility disorders, e.g. megaoesophagus

2. Inflammatory disorders, e.g. oesophagitis, gastro-oesophageal reflux

3. Obstructive lesions, e.g. vascular ring abnormalities, foreign bodies, stricture.[1]

In cases of many pharyngeal or oesophageal disorders it is initially important to differentiate whether the animal is regurgitating or vomiting. Vomiting is characterized as the forceful expulsion of digested, bile-stained food, whilst regurgitation involves a less forceful casting-up of tubular, bile-free, undigested food.[1] Poor body condition (BCS 1/5 or 2/5) is commonly evident, and when present in young animals, those affected will be dramatically smaller than their litter mates. A full history and physical examination needs to be conducted by the veterinary surgeon. Secondary aspiration pneumonia can be evident and is characterized by crackles and bronchovesicular sounds on auscultation.

Feeding an animal with pharyngeal or oesophageal disorders

The feeding of animals with pharyngeal or oesophageal disorders needs to reflect the BSC of the animal. As previously stated, these animals tend to be debilitated due to malnutrition. Foods with greater than 25% DM fat, and energy densities in excess of 4.8 kcal/g DM are recommended.[1] Care should be taken in animals suffering from oesophagitis with gastric reflux. This is due to diets high in fat delaying gastric emptying, which reduces lower oesophageal sphincter pressure, which in turn promotes reflux of food and gastric secretions into the oesophagus. Protein and other nutrients (vitamins and minerals) need to be of an adequate level for the particular requirement of the individual. Highly digestible foods should be used, and feeding little and often can also be of benefit.

Most important is the form in which the food is delivered to the animal. Food consistency plays an important role in the management of pharyngeal and oesophageal disorders. Foods made into a gruel consistency will benefit animals suffering from obstructions, lesions and/or oesophagitis. Oesophageal performance in animals suffering from megaoesophagus can improve when they are fed dry foods or moist foods formed into a bolus. This is due to the swallowing reflex being stimulated by the specific texture. When feeding animals with megaoesophagus, the food should be placed on a raised level. In most cases trial and error is required in order to determine a diet consistency that best suits the animal.

Exocrine pancreatic insufficiency (EPI)

EPI describes a lack of pancreatic enzymes (lipase and amylase) in the gut lumen resulting in steatorrhoea and weight loss. When lipases are absent from the array of brush border enzymes, secondary damage to the small intestine and small intestinal bacterial overgrowth (SIBO) can occur. These complications can further aggravate the malabsorption of nutrients. EPI occurs commonly in young dogs as a congenital abnormality, but may also develop as a sequela to acute or chronic pancreatitis. EPI is rare in cats, but has been reported in both the juvenile and acquired forms.

The nutritional aims include:

- providing a highly digestible diet
- supplementation of exocrine pancreatic enzymes within each meal
- providing sufficient calories and nutrients in the diet to support the particular lifestage of the animal – these may have to be higher than calculated due to the changes in digestion and metabolism.

Clinical nutrition

Fat

Effective treatment of EPI involves the use of pancreatic enzyme supplementation. There are many available on the market, the most effective being in the forms of powders that can be sprinkled onto the diet prior to ingestion. A low-fat highly digestible diet is recommended as a starting point in EPI and is particularly valuable if there is persistent SIBO. The dry matter digestibility of these diets needs to be greater than 90%. There is no reason that once the dog has reached its optimal weight and condition that it cannot return to a good-quality lifestage diet with the use of the pancreatic enzymes. Some larger dogs may find it difficult to achieve a high enough calorific intake on a low-fat diet.

Carbohydrates

In order to help resolve SIBO soluble fibre in the diet is important, as it will help to promote normalization of the gastrointestinal flora. Large amounts of fibre in the diet, however, especially insoluble fibre, will decrease the digestibility of the diet. The diet should contain no more than 2% on a dry matter basis. The use of prebiotics in these cases can prove to be advantageous.

Proteins

Protein levels for animals suffering from EPI need to be in an adequate supply, as protein metabolism for energy is utilized if insufficient fat for this requirement is absorbed. If the diet has a good carbohydrate level, excessive protein quantities would not be required, and the amount should reflect that for the particular lifestage of the animal.

Vitamins and minerals

When any malassimilation or malabsorption is present, supplementation with micronutrients should be considered. When gastrointestinal fat absorption is impaired, so is the solubilization and absorption of the fat-soluble vitamins. The fat-soluble vitamins A and D can be administered intramuscularly, and vitamin K should also be supplemented if coagulopathies are detected in the dog or cat.

Folate and cobalamin/B_{12} levels are also of concern in the cat and dog suffering from EPI. The absence of pancreatic bicarbonate secretion in EPI may reduce intestinal luminal pH and the affinity of cobalamin for intrinsic factor. If SIBO is present the gut microflora may consume the dietary cobalamin before it is able to be absorbed. Folate deficiencies have been shown to inhibit pancreatic exocrine function in rats, and therefore if any deficiencies are present, supplementation with parenteral folate is recommended.

Feeding an animal with EPI

On diagnosis of EPI an initial transition to a highly digestible, low-fat diet is beneficial. This will aid in the normalization of the gut transit times, absorption of nutrients and gastrointestinal flora. Daily administration of pre- and probiotics will also aid in the re-establishment of normal gastrointestinal flora populations. Dogs presenting with EPI tend always to be underweight, and weight gain needs to be monitored.

Even after the animal has reached its ideal bodyweight, it may be necessary to offer the calculated basal energy requirement (BER) plus 20% to allow for the persistent degree of malabsorption in patients with EPI. All patients with EPI should be fed multiple small meals per day with pancreatic enzyme supplementation in order to improve digestibility, dietary overload and osmotic diarrhoea. It is

Key points

- The diet must be supplied predosed with pancreatic enzymes.
- The diet must provide adequate nutrients for the lifestage of the individual, with additional calories to compensate for inadequate absorption.
- The diet provided needs to be ideally highly digestible and low in fat.

CASE STUDY 12.1

A Cavalier King Charles spaniel was presented to a nursing clinic with persistent but intermittent diarrhoea and chronic weight loss. A full nutritional history was taken, as a veterinary surgeon had previously clinically examined the dog a week earlier. After consulting with the veterinary surgeon, a full haematology and biochemistry blood test was performed, including B_{12}/cobalamin and folate, along with faecal analysis (Table 12.3).

The low B_{12}/cobalamin and trypsin-like immunoreactivity (TLI) are both consistent with distal small intestinal disease and EPI. The low albumin levels can be an acute-phase response to inflammation, or may reflect gastrointestinal losses. The high levels of starch in the faecal sample suggest the occurrence of poor digestion. The veterinary surgeon diagnosed the dog as having EPI. Pancreatic supplements were initiated with a low-fat, highly digestible diet, along with antibiotics because of the increased white blood cell count. Weight checks were performed in order to monitor the animal's weight gain to an optimal weight. Once this had been achieved, the dog was changed from a prescription diet to a commercial lifestage diet, due to financial implications. Again, the dog was monitored in nursing clinics for weight and to gain history on any digestive problems that could have arisen from the change in diet.

Table 12.3 **Blood biochemistry and haematology results for Case Study 12.1**

Profile	Levels	Normal ranges
Total protein	56 g/l	54.0–77.0
Albumin	23 g/l	25.0–37.0
Globulin	33 g/l	25.0–52.0
RBC	6.10×10^{12}/l	5.0–8.5
Hb	14.2 g/dl	12.0–18.0
HCT	40.2%	37.0–55.0
MCV	66.0 fl	60.0–80.0
MCH	23.3 pg	19.0–26.0
MCHC	35.4 g/dl	31.5–37.0
Platelets	Giant platelets observed	
WBC	20.74×10^9/l	6.0–15.0
Neutrophils	13.69×10^9/l	3.0–11.5
Bands	1.24×10^9/l	0.0–0.3
Lymphocytes	4.77×10^9/l	1.0–4.8
Monocytes	0.41×10^9/l	0.0–1.3
Eosinophils	0.62×10^9/l	0.0–1.25
Nucleated RBCs	0.62×10^9/l	0.0–4.0
B_{12}	176 ng/l	240–440
Folate	6.7 µg/l	5.0–15.0
TLI	0.4 ng/ml	5.0–40.0

RBC, red blood cell/red blood (cell) count; Hb, haemoglobin; HCT, haematocrit; MCV, mean cell volume; MCH, mean cell haemoglobin; MCHC, mean cell haemoglobin concentration; WBC, white blood (cell) count; TLI, trypsin-like immunoreactivity.

more beneficial for the enzymic supplements to be added to the diet at least 5 minutes prior to consumption. Capsules should always be opened and sprinkled over the diet.

Pancreatitis

The exocrine pancreas is highly responsive to changes in nutritional substrates present within the diet. When the pancreas becomes inflamed, symptoms such as depression, anorexia, vomiting, diarrhoea and displays of abdominal pain can present. Pancreatitis, whether in an acute or chronic form, is a common occurrence seen in veterinary practice. Pancreatitis is exceptionally painful and requires analgesia as its primary treatment. This is due to the proteolytic enzymes being activated in situ, resulting in autodigestion. There are many factors that can predispose to pancreatitis, including breed, age, gender, neuter status and body condition.

Treatment of pancreatitis involves consideration of the following factors:

- Treatment/removal of the initial cause.
- Fluid therapy, in order to maintain hydration and electrolyte levels. Plasma may be required in severe cases.
- Analgesia. Non-steroidal anti-inflammatory drugs (NSAIDs) are best avoided in these cases due to the gastric and renal side effects. A non-ulcerogenic NSAID could be considered in chronic cases.
- The nutritional status of the animal needs to be considered. On a short-term basis should the animal be starved, tube fed or use made of total parenteral nutrition (TPN)? There is currently conflicting evidence to support each. Thought should also be given to long-term dietary management.
- Symptomatic treatment with anti-emetics, antibiotics and anti-ulcer medication as necessary to prevent complications. Use of broad-spectrum antibiotics is twofold: first to combat any infection that might be present; and secondly to protect against septicaemia caused by bacterial translocation.
- In cats hyperglycaemia is often noted, but can be mild and transient, although in some cases diabetes mellitus can develop and may require insulin therapy.

The aims of clinical nutrition are:

- to provide sufficient calories and nutrients to the body without overloading the pancreas
- preventing the possibility of bacterial translocation from the gastrointestinal tract and intestinal atrophy.

Clinical nutrition

Fat

Fat in the diet delays gastric emptying, which can in turn promote vomiting in the dog and cat. The delay in gastric emptying is a significant cause of upper gastrointestinal signs in the dog, including abdominal discomfort, nausea and vomiting. Preventing or inhibiting the release of pancreatic enzymes that aid in digestion of fats is an essential component of treatment. For long-term management, feeding a low-fat diet with or without the use of pancreatic enzymes can reduce postprandial pain. The restriction of fat content of the diet in cats is not as vital as with dogs, but the fat should still be of a highly digestible nature.

Carbohydrates

As the fat content in the diet needs to be reduced yet highly digestible, the carbohydrate content must provide a greater contribution to the metabolizable energy (ME) content of the diet. The carbohydrates present in the diet must be easily digestible, as digestion and absorption may be adversely affected in all cases of gastrointestinal upset.

Vitamins and minerals

Guidelines for vitamin and mineral levels are the same as for the corresponding lifestage. If large volumes of vomiting or diarrhoea are present then care should be taken, as excessive amounts of the water-soluble vitamins can be lost. When feeding an exceptionally low-fat diet, the quantity of fat-soluble vitamins can also be reduced. As some of these vitamins are required in fat metabolism it is important that these losses are replaced.

Hypokalaemia is particularly common in animals suffering from pancreatitis, and can be severe and life-threatening. If vomiting or diarrhoea is present then monitoring of electrolyte balance needs to occur, as it should with any animal receiving intravenous fluid therapy. Oral supplementation may be required.

Supplements

The use of exocrine pancreatic enzymes in cases of acute pancreatitis is starting to become commonplace in veterinary practice. Even if the animal is not displaying clinical symptoms of exocrine pancreatic insufficiency (EPI), these enzymes have an important part to play. Addition of the enzymes to the meal at least 5 minutes prior to feeding has proven to reduce postprandial pain, and does help to ease the pancreas back into work after a period of 'rest'.

Feeding a pancreatic patient

Current dietary therapy for dogs suffering from acute pancreatitis is nil-by-mouth until the clinical symptoms stop, and in some practices this can be up to 5–7 days. Recent evidence has shown that nil-by-mouth in these cases has little benefit to the animal. Very short-term rest (48 hours) is still indicated to allow pancreatic rest in acute pancreatic cases, but for no longer. For any cases that require starving for over 48 hours total parenteral nutrition must be provided, alongside very small amounts of nutrition being given by mouth (microenteral nutrition). The oral nutritional support is required to prevent gastroduodenal ulceration, bacterial translocation from the gut and septicaemia. Small amounts of watered-down baby rice or cottage cheese can be used before moving on to a commercial low-fat, highly digestible diet. Baby rice is the food of choice in these cases, and Table 12.4 demonstrates a typical nutrient analysis.

In cats, nutrition is generally supplied by enteral means (gastrostomy feeding tube), in order to avoid hepatic lipidosis. There is no clinical evidence that this type of nutrition exacerbates the course of acute pancreatitis. There is also evidence that enteral support is superior to parenteral support as described above. Oral intake in cats should only be restricted if persistent vomiting is occurring, and then for as short a time as possible.

Dietary long-term control of pancreatitis is vital, but initially confirmation of the presence of hyperlipidaemia needs to be obtained. Those dogs

Table 12.4 **Typical analysis of baby rice**

Nutrient	Per 100 g (as fed)
Fat	0.8 g
Fibre	1.5 g
Carbohydrates (as sugars)	85.6 g
Protein	8 g

suffering from pancreatitis with associated hyper-lipidaemia will need to be maintained on a different diet than those without. If the lipid levels in the bloodstream are within normal levels then a highly digestible low-fat diet can be used. If hyperlipidaemia is concurrent then a low-fat diet is required again, but these types of diets can have a corresponding high-fibre content, thus reducing digestibility. This can be advantageous as the majority of

dogs that suffer from hyperlipidaemia tend to be overweight and can benefit from this type of diet.

Weight control is important in these cases, as a major predisposing factor is obesity and being fed high-fat treats. By altering the diet in order to reduce fat content, most animals will gradually lose weight but this does need to be monitored regularly.

Key points

- Analgesia is the most important aspect of treating any animal with pancreatitis.
- Use of minimal enteral nutrition in order to prevent bacterial translocation.
- Use of exogenous pancreatic enzymes.

CASE STUDY 12.2

An 8-year-old cocker spaniel was presented with cranial abdominal pain and vomiting. Blood biochemistries identified a rise in amylase and lipase profiles. The dog was diagnosed with acute pancreatitis. Initial management was analgesia, intravenous fluid therapies, anti-emetics and nil-by-mouth. The dog had a BCS of 5, and showed hyperlipidaemia on blood sampling. The vomiting stopped 24 hours after initiation of the medical therapies, and the dog was placed on small portions of baby rice and cottage cheese (with exogenous enzymes) for the next 24 hours. No further vomiting was experienced, so the dog was started on a low-fat, highly digestible diet (again with exogenous pancreatic enzymes). The dog was later discharged from the practice, but its long-term dietary plan was different from the short-term dietary plan. Long-term, because of the hyperlipidaemia, the dog will require a low-fat diet, but one that is also high in fibre. This will also aid in weight reduction. In pancreatic cases the presence of hyperlipidaemia will dictate the long-term dietary plan of choice. Exogenous pancreatic enzymes were continued for 14 days.

EQUINE

Colic

Colic is a term used to describe abdominal pain, and is not a diagnosis in itself – it is a clinical symptom. Colic can be caused through a multitude of different aetiologies, though many colics involve the presence of a thick sticky mass of fermenting feed, or a compacted mass of roughage, in the stomach or intestines.

Types of colic

- Spasmodic (an increase in bowel movements due to a sudden change in diet, work or consuming chilled food or water, or frosty grass).
- Foal colic (caused by meconium retention).
- Sand.
- Large intestinal impactions.
- Ileal impactions (ileus).
- Colic associated with torsion, twists and rotations.
- Gas or flatulent colic.

Some of these types of colic will be discussed separately later in the chapter, especially those relating to diet.

Oral and dietary treatments
When a horse presents with abdominal pain (colic) feed should be removed until the cause has been determined by the veterinary surgeon. Clean fresh water should be available to the horse at all times. General treatment has the objective of preventing rupture or displacement of some part of the gastrointestinal tract; this is achieved by controlling pain and tympany, evacuation of the bowels, stopping bacterial fermentation and re-establishment

of the normal process of peristalsis. In cases where fermentation has occurred, removing food components that are highly fermentable from the diet is required. This tends to be those with high sugar contents, such as products coated with molasses. Where impactions are present, oral fluids, including solutions of electrolytes and glucose should be used, but solid foods should not be consumed until the impaction is passed. Use of soapy enemas has proven to be useful in cases of colonic impaction in foals. In adult horses enemas of 9–13 l with or without the addition of mineral oil as a lubricant can be utilized.[13]

Rehydration of the horse is essential, both orally, if no reflux is present, and intravenously. When severe impactions are present, the dose estimated to be appropriate for a 500-kg horse is 6 l of fluid every 2 hours, given via an indwelling nasogastric tube.[13] Once gastrointestinal function has been restored, mashes of bran are the diet of choice for the first 24–48 hours, as they act as an osmotic laxative. The next stage is to gradually introduce hay, along with concentrate mashes, or short grazing spells. In cases where prolonged dysfunction of the gastrointestinal tract has occurred, partial or total parenteral nutrition may be required. The use of short chopped forage should be avoided, as it has been linked to an increased disposition to ileal obstructions.[13]

In some cases surgical intervention may be required. In these cases nutritional support will depend on the initial cause of the abdominal pain and the type of surgery required.

Key points

- A poor diet is a major determinant of the risk of colic in horses.
- A concentrate diet has a higher risk factor than that of forage.
- Dietary change leads to an increased risk of colic. The equine GIT can adapt to change, but only slowly.
- Seasonal patterns of colic are consistent with dietary risk factors.[14]

Diarrhoea

Acute diarrhoea

In the majority of cases, acute diarrhoea is caused by salmonella infection, precipitated by stress factors, and particularly by infection of strongyle parasites.

Salmonella may be transmitted to foals by adults that are symptomatic carriers.[13] All cases of acute-onset diarrhoea are linked with an acute loss of fluids and electrolytes, especially potassium, sodium and chloride. Treatment involves rehydration of the animal and correction of electrolyte losses. In cases of severe diarrhoea, potassium losses can become severe, resulting in weakness of skeletal and smooth muscles, tremors, and in cases of severe potassium depletion recumbency, cyanosis and eventually respiratory and heart failure.[13] Correction of potassium levels should be carried out either orally or via nasogastric intubation. This is due to the administration of potassium intravenously having the potential to cause cardiac complications.

Chronic diarrhoea

Horses suffering from chronic diarrhoea often suffer from protein-losing gastroenteropathy (PLGE).[15] This is due to a loss in the integrity of the mucosa, or through lymphangiectasia. These cases often show clinical signs of weight loss, anorexia, lethargy, pyrexia and colic. Often energy, mineral and vitamin malnutrition also occurs. Horses should be fed ad libitum hay, preferable alfalfa hay due to the increase in protein and mineral levels, alongside a high-protein–energy concentrate, and a mineral and vitamin supplement. In some cases a reduction in fibre content may be required, as some horses can have an impaired fibre digestion.[15] A diet of choice would have a decreased proportion of fibre and an increased proportion of grains and concentrates in order to maintain optimal weight and BCS.

Colitis sufferers tend to suffer concurrently from severe electrolyte imbalances. Acidotic animals will require intensive corrective fluid therapy, and should be offered fresh water alongside an electrolyte solution. Their diets should consist solely of grass hay for approximately 2 weeks during convalescence.[15] This is due to a reduction in the normal

GIT microflora. Because of this, supplementation of the B vitamin complex may be required. The use of pre- and probiotics is often advocated in these cases, but the benefits of pasture should not be forgotten in aiding the normalization of GIT microflora.

Foal heat diarrhoea

Foal heat diarrhoea usually occurs at the time of the dam's first postpartum oestrus. It is usually self-limiting secretory diarrhoea. If prolonged, fluid and electrolyte replacement should occur.

Flatulent colic

Flatulent or gas colic can be as a result of an impaction or obstruction, and will cause extreme pain in the horse. Where gastric tympany occurs, decompression with a nasogastric tube is required immediately. Ruptures and volvulus can occur in response to the horse's violent reactions to the pain. Gastric tympany usually becomes evident 4–6 hours postprandially.[13] Where impactions have been the initiating cause, treatment to facilitate the passing or removing of the obstructing ingesta should be made. Gas colic can result from a rich diet of highly fermentable products such as cereals, lush legumes or from consumption of grass cuttings. Fluids and laxatives should also be utilized in order to increase transit time of these food items through the GIT.

Gastric impaction

Gastric impaction is uncommon in the horse, but can be diagnosed as a cause of colic. Diagnosis can be made through the use of endoscopy, or laparotomy. Treatments involve aiding in facilitating the passage of the ingesta. This can be achieved through nasogastric intubation to hydrate the impaction with water and laxatives. During gastric lavage some of the material can also be removed. In surgical cases saline can be injected into the stomach, and the impaction massaged. Gastric impactions could be associated with the ingestion of coarse roughage and an inadequate water intake, although there is no scientific evidence to support this theory.[13]

Gastric ulceration

Gastric ulcers are most highly prevalent amongst racehorses in training. Horses can present with poor performance, recurrent colic, poor appetite and weight loss. Risk factors for gastric ulceration include stress, drug administration (NSAIDs), high-concentrate/low-roughage diets, periods of fasting and exercise.[16] Where food is withheld for periods of time (several hours) the pH of the gastric fluid can decrease to 2 and below. In horses receiving ad libitum (free choice) timothy hay, the gastric fluid has a higher pH of 3. It has been determined that equine gastric ulcers are not caused by *Helicobacter pylori* bacteria, which is a common cause of ulcers in humans.[17] Dehydration and reduced water intake may further increase the ill effects of acid on the stomach.

Management modifications that aid in removing or reducing these stress factors are important. Increasing the level of roughage and decreased periods of fasting should be a vital element in any management regimen. The type of roughage used appears to have beneficial effects. The mineral content (especially calcium) appears to have an effect on gastric activity. Grains and pelleted concentrates also increase the level of production of gastrin in comparison to hay fed alone.[17]

Intestinal impactions

Ileal impactions

The ileum is the most common site of impactions of the small intestine, though impactions of the jejunum and duodenum have been reported.[18] Aetiologies of ileal impactions are unknown, but dietary implications have been made. The feeding of coastal Bermuda hay, with its fine, high-roughage consistency may predispose to these impactions. Other causes of ileal impaction include ileal hypertrophy, mesenteric vascular thrombotic disease, tapeworm infections and ascarid infections; though all are less common than intraluminal feed impactions.[18] Treatment of these cases is usually through surgical interventions. Medical therapies used in the first instance include gastric decompression, intravenous fluids, analgesics and intensive monitoring.

Where impactions occur, ileus can also result. This is defined as a loss of smooth muscle action with its peristaltic movement of digesta.[13] Food and water should be withheld in these cases until the impaction has been resolved, as further ingesta can aggravate gastric distension.

Large intestinal impactions

Aetiologies of large intestinal impactions are similar to those within the small intestine. *Salmonella* spp. have also been associated with inflammatory conditions and therefore may predispose to colon impactions.[18] Impactions of the caecum respond favourably to medical therapy. Food should be withheld in all cases of impaction, but water should be allowed if there is no nasogastric reflux present. Large volumes of fluid need to be administered for severe cases, up to three times maintenance; this can equate to 6 l of fluid per 500-kg horse every 2 hours. Administration is achieved via a nasogastric tube.[18] In mild cases one to two times maintenance is required. Laxatives should also be used in order to hydrate the impacted ingesta. Once impactions have resolved, feeding of the animal should be resumed, but slowly. Mashes should be utilized in the first 24–48 hours; once the horse has responded well to this diet hay and grain can be introduced, again slowly.

Large colon impactions usually occur at the two sites of narrowing within the large colon; the pelvic flexure and transverse colon.[18] Retropulsive contractions also occur within these regions, and can exacerbate impactions. These cases require initial therapy as with caecal impactions; administration of water (if no nasogastric reflux) and laxatives. Surgical intervention in these cases may also be required.

Sand impactions

Impactions of sand usually occur when the horse is grazed in areas where the soil contains large amounts of sand, or when drinking from sandy-bottomed streams. Ingested sand settles to the bottom of the colon, where accumulation and obstructions can occur. Treatments are made through the administration of fluids and laxatives, the most commonly used laxative being psyllium hydrophilic mucilloid, administered at a dose of 400 g/500 kg BW every 6 hours until the impaction has resolved. The laxative therapy should then continue at 400 g/500 kg BW daily for 3 weeks in order to remove the remaining sand from the colon.

Oesophageal impactions (choke)

Oesophageal impactions or choke can be induced through a number of different reasons, but immediate veterinary attention should be sought for these cases, alongside a withdrawal of food. In many cases the obstruction will clear itself; in more severe cases, intubation after sedation, and a warm water lavage with external massage is required to help dislodge the impaction. Factors disposing to choke include:

- *Greediness.* Consumption of the diet too quickly can lead to reduction in saliva in the throat. In these cases encouraging the horse to eat more slowly is required.

- *Poor dentition.* Horses with poor dentition cannot masticate their diets as proficiently as those with good dentition, resulting in the diet components not being chewed for long enough and a consequent reduction in the quantity of saliva produced. Dental treatment is required; the horse may also benefit from soak feeds.

- *Inadequate water.* In cases where water deprivation occurs, water is drawn from the intestinal tract and saliva production in order to maintain homeostasis. Rehydration with fluids is required prior to feeding.

- *Foreign bodies.* Any foreign body within the oesophagus will increase the risk of choke, as the food bolus is unable to pass through into the stomach in the correct manner.

Once the impaction has been resolved, feeding should consist of soaked feeds, little and often with free access to water.

References

1. Buffington CAT, Holloway C, Abood SK. Manual of veterinary dietetics. Missouri: Elsevier Saunders; 2004.
2. Krempels D, Cotter M, Stanzione G. Ileus in domestic rabbits. Exotic DVM 2000; 2(4):19–21.
3. Battersby I, Harvey A. Differential diagnosis and treatment of acute diarrhoea in the dog and cat. In Practice 2006; 28:480–488.
4. McCann T, Simpson JW. Approach to the management of diarrhoea. UK Vet 2006; 11(6):30–37.
5. Davenport DJ, Remillard RL, Simpson KW, et al. Gastrointestinal and exocrine pancreatic disease. In: Hand MS, Thatcher CD, Remillard RL, et al., eds. Small animal clinical nutrition. 4th edn. Missouri: Mark Morris Institute; 2000:725–810.
6. Elwood CM. Risk factors for gastric dilation in Irish setter dogs. J Small Anim Pract 1998; 39:185–190.
7. King C. Gastrointestinal tract and stasis in the rabbit. VN Times 2005; (Nov):19.
8. Ragni RA. GDV: preventing the nightmare is best. Veterinary Times 31 October 2005:6–7.
9. Brewer NR, Cruise LJ. Physiology. In: Manning PJ, Ringer DH, Newcomer CE, eds. The biology of the laboratory rabbit. San Diego: Academic Press; 1994:65.
10. Watson PJ. Managing canine pancreatitis. BSAVA Congress 2005 Scientific Proceedings. 2005:97–99.
11. Carpenter JW, Mashima TY, Gentz EJ. Caring for rabbits: an overview and formulary. Vet Med 1995; 90:340–364.
12. Williams DA. The exocrine pancreas. In: Kelly N, Wills J, eds. BSAVA manual of companion animal nutrition and feeding. Gloucester: BSAVA Publications; 1996:161–166.
13. Frape DF. Equine nutrition and feeding. 2nd edn. Oxford: Blackwell Science; 1998.
14. Proudman C. Dietary risk factors for equine colic: what's the evidence? Proceedings of the Dodson and Horrell 5th International Feeding Conference. 2005:19–28.
15. Harris PA, Frape DL, Jeffcott LB, et al. Equine nutrition and metabolic disease. In: Higgins AJ, Wright IM, eds. The equine manual. London: Saunders; 1995:123–185.
16. Steel N. Equine gastroscopy: What do veterinarians need to know? Veterinary Times 17 October 2005:8.
17. Pagan JD. Gastric ulcers in horses: A widespread but manageable disease. In: Pagan JD, Geor RJ, eds. Advances in equine nutrition II. Kentucky: Kentucky Equine Research; 2000:387–391.
18. Eades SC, Booth AJ, Hansen TO, et al. The gastrointestinal and digestive system. In: Higgins AJ, Wright IM, eds. The equine manual. London: Saunders; 1995:453–539.

13
Hepatic disorders

Hepatobiliary disease

The role of the liver in the body is critical in maintaining homeostasis and the removal of waste products that have accumulated within the body. The liver is essential in the production of proteins and deamination of excessive unrequired proteins. Understanding the functioning of the organ is essential in designing a diet relating to the clinical symptoms that the animal is exhibiting. The liver can be damaged in a number of different ways, from infection and hepatic encephalopathy as an adjunct to medical therapies and from toxins. Congenital abnormalities such as portal systemic shunts will also affect the way in which the liver functions. Analysis of laboratory results and other diagnostic means will enable the practitioner to identify where the damage is occurring within the liver. Delayed recovery from general anaesthesia may be the first indication of compromised liver function. Nutritional management of hepatobiliary disease is usually directed at clinical manifestations of the disease rather than the specific cause itself. The aims of nutritional management are:

- maintaining the normal metabolic processes
- avoiding toxic by-product accumulation
- correcting any electrolyte disturbances
- providing substrates that support hepatocellular regeneration and repair.

There is no one 'ideal' liver disease treatment or diet. The dietary needs of the patient require a good understanding of what you are trying to achieve and the individual animal's needs. A palatable high-quality protein diet, supplemented with zinc,

B vitamins and antioxidants should be fed.[1] Protein should not be restricted unless it is essential to control encephalopathy.[2] Malnutrition is a very common feature of chronic hepatic disease, and correct nutrition for each individual patient is important to help regulate the hormonal derangement that results from hepatic injury.

Clinical nutrition
Protein
The maintenance of a positive nitrogen balance is important for the preservation of body condition and protein synthesis. Protein malnutrition is common in patients with chronic liver disease, where the clinical manifestations include weight loss, loss of muscle tissue and hypoalbuminaemia. Protein intake needs to be finely balanced; in some dogs the protein requirements may exceed those of normal maintenance requirements because of the increased protein turnover and the demands of hepatocellular regeneration. A moderate restriction of protein levels is not always recommended, and the quality (biological value) of the proteins should be increased. This is recommended because they fulfil the animal's needs with minimal production of nitrogenous waste. Studies have shown in human patients with hepatic failure that the nitrogen balance can be improved if the diet is divided into small, frequent meals.[2]

Dairy products (cottage cheese, milk) or eggs are of excellent benefit, probably related to factors such as the relatively high ratio of carbohydrates to protein, their influence on intestinal transit and colonic pH, as well as the differing amino acid composition. Fibre of soya origin has been shown to provide an excellent source of dietary fibre that reduces ammonia production and absorption in the colon and assists ammonia elimination in the faeces.[3]

One of the roles of the liver is a protein regulatory event, including degradation of the essential amino acids (including the aromatic amino acids (AAA), but not the branched-chain amino acids (BCAA)) and some of the non-essential amino acids. Dogs and other omnivores are able to downregulate the activities of protein degradation when minimal dietary protein is consumed; cats are not able to do this. Plasma amino acid concentrations differ depending on the type of hepatic failure. In the normal healthy animal AAA (i.e. tyrosine, phenylalanine and tryptophan) are effectively extracted from the portal circulation and metabolized by the liver. Reduced hepatic function is associated with an increase in circulating AAA. Conversely the plasma concentrations of BCAA (i.e. leucine, isoleucine and valine) and most other amino acids are reduced due to an increased rate of metabolizing by muscle and adipose tissue. The ratio between AAA and BCAA can be used in order to evaluate the liver function. In healthy dogs the ratio between BCAA and AAA ranges between 3.0 to 4.0.[4] This ratio can be reduced to 1.0 or less in dogs with portosystemic vascular anomalies and chronic hepatitis. Other factors such as increased levels of insulin, glucagons and catecholamines are thought to contribute to the altered amino acid metabolism seen in these patients. Alterations in this ratio have also been implicated in the pathogenesis of hepatic encephalopathy. Hence BCAA-enriched solutions have been used in human nutritional support for many years in those patients suffering from chronic hepatic disease and hepatic encephalopathy.

Carbohydrates and fats
Non-protein calories should come from highly digestible carbohydrate and fat sources. The fat level in the diet should not be restricted unless there is clinical evidence of steatorrhoea.

Vitamins and minerals
The requirement of vitamins and minerals within the diet is dependent on the causal problem with the liver. Copper levels should be restricted because of accumulation within the liver, and this is discussed further below. Vitamins that are produced within the liver should be supplemented, as deficiencies are common, as is deficiency of zinc. Because of the oxidative cell damage, which is correlated with the severity of liver disease, antioxidants should also be supplemented.

Copper-associated hepatotoxicosis in dogs
Bedlington terriers can often develop copper storage disease and subsequently hepatitis and cirrhosis. Statistics state that roughly 25% of Bedlington terriers are affected and another 50% are carriers. Some other breeds have also been affected, namely the West Highland white terriers and Doberman

pinschers. Copper-associated hepatotoxicosis is caused by an inherited autosomal recessive trait that results is impaired biliary excretion of copper. Thus diets for these dogs need to have a reduction in the copper levels. Supplements containing copper should also be avoided. Homemade diets should not contain liver, shellfish and organ meats, which are all high in copper content.

The role of copper in hepatic diseases in other breeds of dogs is less clear. There are theories that elevated hepatic copper concentrations precede liver damage, whereas others contend that the excess hepatic copper results from faulty copper excretion caused by chronic cholestasis. A third theory is that elevated levels are antecedent to the disease and are incidental to disease progression.[4] Anti-inflammatory agents, such as prednisolone, can be beneficial in the management of chronic hepatitis in Bedlington terriers and West Highland white terriers.

The nutritional aims of managing patients with copper-associated hepatotoxicosis are:

- to decrease further absorption of copper from the gastrointestinal tract
- to enhance copper excretion.

Portal systemic shunts (PSS) and hepatic encephalopathy (HE)

Portal systemic shunts (PSS) are vascular communications between the portal and systemic venous systems. This communication allows access of portal blood to the systemic circulation without passing through the liver. Congenital PSS are most common and are inherited. They may either be intrahepatic (large breeds such as Irish wolfhound and Burmese mountain dog) or extrahepatic (medium and toy breeds, such as Yorkshire terrier, Cairn terrier and Dachshund). Stunted growth or failure to gain weight can occur in these animals. Acquired PSS form in response to portal hypertension caused by fibrosis and chronic cirrhosis.[2] As a result of inadequate hepatic clearance of toxins and altered liver function, hepatic encephalopathy can result. Ammonium urate and other purine uroliths can also occur due to the high urinary excretion of ammonia and uric acid.

Shunting results in nutritional depletion of the liver as well as failed delivery of substrates to the liver for degradation and metabolism. Hepatic encephalopathy is a complex metabolic disorder, which is characterized by abnormal mental status. There are many factors that can precipitate HE, which are detailed in Box 13.1.

The nutritional aims for managing patients with hepatic encephalopathy include:

- reducing dietary protein
- changing intestinal flora
- decreasing intestinal transit time.

Soluble or fermentable fibre in the diet, such as cellulose and lactulose, aids animals suffering from liver dysfunction as it helps reduce the side effects of deamination of proteins. Lactulose is a synthetic disaccharide that is hydrolysed into volatile/short-chain fatty acids in the colon. The change in the lumen pH traps the ammonia as ammonium ions, which are removed in the faeces. There is also the beneficial effect that colonic bacteria use the increasing nitrogen in reproduction and growth, whilst also inhibiting ammonia generation by colonic bacteria through a process known as catabolite repression.[5]

Insoluble or non-fermentable fibre is also an important constituent in the diet of animals suffering from hepatic disease. Constipation is a predisposing factor for the development of encephalopathy since it increases the contact time for colonic bacteria to act on the faeces and produce ammonia.

Box 13.1 Factors precipitating hepatic encephalopathy (HE)

- High-protein meal
- GI bleeding or ingestion of blood
- Transfusion of stored blood
- Constipation
- Azotaemia
- Metabolic alkalosis
- Hypokalaemia
- Dietary methionine
- Catabolism/hypermetabolism
- Sedatives/anaesthetics

Vitamins and minerals

Vitamin E is a superb antioxidant and may be cytoprotective, especially in copper toxicity, because of the effect it has in protecting against lipid peroxidation. Vitamin K supplementation may become a necessity if clotting times are prolonged, especially prior to hepatic biopsies being taken. The vitamin K stores within the liver are limited and become rapidly depleted, although the function of synthesis of the prothrombin-complex clotting factors is always lost before the storage of vitamin K is depleted. The other fat-soluble vitamins, A and D, should not be supplemented, as vitamin A can cause hepatic damage and vitamin D can cause calcification within the tissues.

The level of calorific intake determines the requirements for the water-soluble vitamins. Thus if anorexia is present the requirement is low, but when nutrition intake increases, the water-soluble vitamins are required in order to replenish coenzymes involved in metabolic processes in the liver and other tissues. As with all animals suffering from polydipsia and polyuria, supplementation with B vitamins is required. Animals suffering from hepatic disease have been recommended to receive a double dose of B vitamins. Vitamin C should not be supplemented as it can increase the tissue damage associated with copper and iron disease.

Choline is essential in the packaging of very low-density lipoprotein (VLDL) in the liver and therefore the exportation of triglycerides. A choline deficiency with concurrent lipolysis may slow down VLDL export and promote hepatic lipid accumulation.[4] Hepatic diets should contain supplementation of choline and L-carnitine, but the efficacy levels are unknown.

There are large amounts of supportive data that zinc deficiency is common in hepatic injury. This is due to a reduction in absorption and an increased loss via the urine. Supplementation of the diet with zinc reduces encephalopathy at an effective rate the same as lactulose.

Feeding a hepatic diet

The aim of the dietary modifications is to meet the animal's daily requirement for nutrients, whilst reducing the metabolic demands placed upon the liver. The calorific needs of the liver should be met with non-protein calories, and the nutritional deficiencies that can occur due to the loss of hepatic function need to be met within the diet.

Frequent feeding of small meals is preferred to ensure optimal assimilation and to limit the entry of dietary protein into the colon. Other complications of liver disease include gastrointestinal ulceration and ascites. If ulceration is known to be present the animal must not go without food.

Idiopathic feline hepatic lipidosis

The incidence rate of feline hepatic lipidosis is unfortunately increasing. Most of these cats are obese and usually present with a history of prolonged anorexia after a stressful event. Hepatic lipidosis is characterized by accumulation of excess triglycerides in the hepatocytes, which results in cholestasis and hepatic dysfunction. This disease may be idiopathic or may develop secondary to some underlying medical problem. Hepatic lipidosis is more commonly seen in cats because of the several special features that make the cat less tolerant of periods of anorexia. Reasons for this include the cat's reduced ability to synthesize arginine when compared with other species. This specific amino acid is an intermediate of the urea cycle, in which ammonia is converted to urea. Its other role is in the production of apoproteins, which are incorporated into VLDL.[1] VLDLs transport triglycerides from the liver to adipose tissue. Any changes in the availability of arginine can result in hyperammonaemia, even when there is minimal hepatic dysfunction, and disturbance to the transportation of triglycerides. Taurine is also required in VLDL production and the conjugation of bile acids. As taurine is also required in larger amounts in the cat, any deficiencies can result in VLDL disturbances. L-Carnitine is also essential in the transportation of long-chain fatty acids into the mitochondria, and is often supplemented in hepatic diets and obesity diets for this very reason, aiding in the mobilization of circulating fats. If any of these supply chains become unbalanced then hepatic lipidosis can occur. Since any disruption in hepatic lipid metabolism can cause lipidosis, it is unlikely that there is a common cause for all cases of feline hepatic lipidosis. Hypokalaemia is present in about 30% of cats with severe hepatic lipidosis; hence electrolyte monitoring is important, as hypokalaemia can prolong anorexia and exacerbate expression of hepatic encephalopathy.[1]

Insulin resistance with subsequent glucose intolerance represents a key metabolic abnormality in all patients with chronic hepatic injury. This can be due to reduced insulin activity from depletion of insulin receptors on the target cells. This is why many cats with hepatic lipidosis are hyperglycaemic. Reduced insulin activity results in activation of triacylglycerol lipase, with consequent hydrolysis of triglycerols, resulting in the increased release of free fatty acids into the circulation from the adipose tissue.

Treatment of feline hepatic lipidosis

Nutrition plays a supportive role in the management of most hepatic diseases, but nutritional therapy is the primary treatment for feline idiopathic hepatic lipidosis. It is a condition that requires vigorous supportive care; this includes intravenous fluids and nutritional support. The provision of an adequate daily energy intake is the cornerstone of successful medical management. This can only be truly achieved through early tube feeding via a nasogastric tube. Force-feeding of the cat or the use of appetite stimulants can work to a degree, but rarely meets the calorific needs of the cat. Food aversion is an exceptionally important component to be considered when tempting anorexic cats, which is why tube feeding is a preferable method. Intravenous feeding (total parenteral feeding) is not recommended unless some enteral nutrition is also being concurrently provided. Parenteral feeding is associated with hepatic steatosis, villus atrophy, fluid and electrolyte imbalances, and an increased incidence of sepsis. Enteral nutrition provides antigenic stimulation to the gut-associated lymphoid tissue (GALT) and stimulates secretion of IgA, which helps to maintain an intact gastrointestinal barrier, in order to prevent bacterial translocation.[1] Other factors that need to be considered in these cases include:

- *Correction of hypokalaemia.* This can be achieved by potassium supplementation through intravenous fluids and oral tube feeding methods.
- *Correction of hyperglycaemia,* and cell intake of calories. Because of glucose intolerance, carbohydrates should not replace the dietary fat.
- *Appropriate protein intake.* Dietary protein intake needs to be adapted to suit the individual patient. It is advised that the protein intake should not be reduced below 20% of calories from this source.

- *Fulfilling energy requirements.* When starting tube feeding a balanced formulation sufficient to meet the cat's resting energy requirements (RER) at its current weight is ideal. In grossly obese cats carrying 35% or more fat, they should be fed at a lower estimated optimal weight rather than their current weight.

Supplements

S-adenosylmethionine (SAMe)

Glutathione is a major antioxidant produced by the liver; its main function is to reduce oxidative damage to the hepatocytes by free radicals. When the liver is compromised there is an increased production of free radicals, and thus the extent of the oxidative stress suffered by hepatocytes is increased. An increased supply of glutathione is required because production is also decreased during hepatic disease. The supply of glutathione is via *S*-adenosylmethionine (SAMe). SAMe initiates three major biochemical pathways: transmethylation, transulphuration and aminopropylation, which all help promote liver health and preserve functioning liver tissue.

Milk thistle

Milk thistle is a herb that contains an active antioxidant bioflavonoid complex known as silymarin.[6] Silymarin stimulates the production of glutathione and glutathione peroxidase (see also Ch. 2 on antioxidants), and has cell-protective properties, especially within the liver.

Equine hepatic disorders

Dietary recommendations for horses with liver dysfunction include the same nutritional ideas as with other companion animals. Recommendations include:

- The daily ration should be divided into at least three meals. This will help reduce the incidence of encephalopathy postprandially.
- Protein levels should be restricted, but of the highest quality available. A 10% protein coarse mix is ideal.
- The branched-chain amino acids isoleucine and valine should be supplemented in the diet (1 g/kg of diet for each).[7]

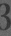

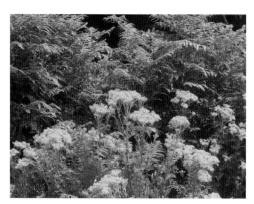

Figure 13.1 Bracken and ragwort have been implicated in the potential to cause liver dysfunction.

- The use of the soluble fibres should be advocated, in order to aid in binding ammonia from the colon and excreting it in the faeces,[8] or for gut bacterial use. Starch levels need to be increased to compensate for the restricted fat and protein levels in the diet. A diet designed for maintenance has ideal starch levels.

- The use of fat supplements is not recommended, though the use of omega-3 oils has been shown to aid in the reduction of inflammatory processes.

- The vitamins E, C and B complex should be supplemented in the diet. Recommendations of 1500 IU/day of vitamin E, 10 g/day of vitamin C, and B vitamins at 1000 mg/kg diet are given. Vitamin E is required due to its antioxidant properties, whilst vitamin C and some of the B complex are synthesized in the liver.

- Suitable pasture should be used; contamination with plants that can exacerbate hepatic dysfunction must be removed (Fig. 13.1).

Key point

- Individual assessment of each animal and the underlying disease process initially needs to be made prior to deciding on diet of choice.

CASE STUDY 13.1

An unstable epileptic Springer spaniel neutered female of 4 years of age has been receiving many medications in order to control her epilepsy. She currently receives phenobarbital, Valium and potassium bromide for the epilepsy. Routine 6-monthly blood tests have resulted in the dog receiving the correct dosage of her medication, but she is also suffering from therapeutic medication-induced hepatitis (Table 13.1). The dog is also predisposed to pancreatitis and has had several acute bouts, and suffers from arthritis and incontinence.

Designing a suitable diet for this dog is difficult due to the different disease processes that are presenting. A low-fat diet is essential because of the pancreatitis, but protein levels also need to be reduced, but of a high biological value. Initially the dog was on a hepatic diet, but the restricted protein levels caused an overall increase in the fat content of the diet. Hyperlipidaemia was also present, but a high-fibre diet was not considered, owing to the effects of the fibre, reducing efficacy of any medications that were being administered.

After consulting one of the food manufacturer's advice lines, it was decided that one of the dermatological diets was the diet of choice. This was due to egg being the protein source (thus providing the highest quality of proteins, for the lowest amount consumed), along with a low-fat concentrate. Animals being administered potassium bromide are advised to consume a low-salt diet. This is due to salts in the diet combining with the potassium bromide, thus reducing the efficacy of the therapy.

Nutraceutical supplements for the arthritis and to support liver function were also added to the diet. Adjunctive therapies of acupuncture and hydrotherapy were also recommended, in order to aid in reducing the quantity of medications that were being administered.

Table 13.1 Biochemistry parameters of case study

Biochemistry	Value	Normal parameters
Total protein	59.7 g/l	54.0–77.0
Albumin	24.4 g/l (low)	25.0–37.0
Total globulin	35.3 g/l	23.0–52.0
Sodium	151 mmol/l	139–154
Potassium	5.70 mmol/l (high)	3.60–5.60
Sodium : potassium	26.49 (low)	27.00–38.00
Chloride	135 mmol/l (high)	105–122
Calcium	2.37 mmol/l	2.30–3.00
Phosphate	1.72 mmol/l (high)	0.80–1.60
Urea	4.6 mmol/l	1.7–7.4
Creatinine	69 µmol/l	0–106
Total bilirubin	1.3 µmol/l	0–16.0
ALKP	7480 U/l (high)	0–50
ALT	141 U/l (high)	0–25
Gamma-GT	15.0 U/l	0.0–27.0
GLDH	7.0 U/l	0.0–10.0
Bile acids	7.2 µmol/l	0.0–10.0
CK	231 U/l (high)	0–190
Cholesterol	10.6 mmol/l (high)	3.8–7.0
Triglycerides	2.22 mmol/l (high)	0.56–1.69
Glucose – random	4.0 mmol/l	2.0–5.5
Amylase	1235 U/l (high)	100–900
Lipase	578 U/l (high)	0–250

ALKP, alkaline phosphatase; ALT, alanine aminotransferase; Gamma-GT, gamma-glutamyl transpeptidase; GLDH, glutamate dehydrogenase; CK, creatine kinase.

References

1. Kuehn NF. Nutritional management of feline hepatic lipidosis. Recent advances in canine and feline nutrition. Volume 3. Iams Nutrition Symposium Proceedings; 2000:333–338.
2. Meyer HP, Rothuizen J. Chronic hepatobiliary disease. In: Kelly N, Wills J, eds. BSAVA manual of companion animal nutrition and feeding. Gloucester: BSAVA Publications; 1996:137–143.
3. Remillard RL, Saker KE. Nutritional management of hepatic conditions. In: Ettinger SJ, Feldman EC, eds. Textbook of veterinary internal medicine. Volume 1. 6th edn. St Louis, Missouri: Elsevier Saunders; 2005:574–577.
4. Roudebush P, Davenport DJ, Dimski DS. Hepatobiliary disease. In: Hand MS, Thatcher CD, Remillard RL, et al., eds. Small animal clinical nutrition. 4th edn. Missouri: Mark Morris Institute; 2000:811–847.
5. Watson PJ. Treatment of chronic liver disease in dogs. Proceedings of Vetoquinol Lecture Tour; 2005.
6. Thorne J. To supplement or not to supplement. Part 3: Antioxidants. VN Times February 2006:10–11.
7. Frape DF. Equine nutrition and feeding. 2nd edn. Oxford: Blackwell Science; 1998.
8. Lakeman N. Faecal ammonium ion concentrations: the benefits of soluble fibre. Dissertation Project. University of the West of England: Hartpury College; 1999.

14
Immune function and cognitive dysfunction

IMMUNE FUNCTION

The interactions between nutrition and immune function are well documented. Any diet that has a nutrient deficiency, whether it is deficient in protein, energy, minerals, vitamins or fats, will impair immune function. Supplements or nutraceuticals that improve immune function are now available commercially. These include both antioxidants and other ingredients that are not traditionally recognized as nutritional requirements of mammals. These compounds may be derived from foods or food ingredients (and include garlic, grape seed extracts, green tea and isoflavones), or from herbs and botanicals (Table 14.1).[1] No specific research has been conducted on companion animals. Most evidence is extrapolated from other species and humans.

COGNITIVE DYSFUNCTION

Cognitive dysfunction describes geriatric behavioural changes that are not solely attributed to a general medical condition, such as infection, organ failure or neoplasm.[2] Other terms such as senile dementia and senile degeneration of the brain are also often used. It should be remembered that cognitive dysfunction should not be considered a normal process of 'getting old'. It is rather a pathological condition that can result from encephalitis, tumours or other structural diseases, metabolic conditions (e.g. hypothyroidism), or be idiopathic in origin.

Nutritional aims when feeding a dog suffering from cognitive dysfunction include:

Table 14.1 **Examples of some dietary supplements and their functions in supporting the immune function**

Food compound	Function in aiding the immune system
Garlic	Augments macrophage and T-cell functions, inhibits tumour growth
Ginseng	Activation of a Th-1 type cellular immunity, enhances bacterial clearance, and has been shown to decrease lung pathology in rats
Grape seed extract	Cytotoxic effect against some cancer cells, and increases the resistance against oxidative stress
Green tea	Ameliorates tumour-related immune dysfunction
Blue-green algae	Increases humoral and cell-mediated immunity. Increases immune cell translocation and activity
Echinacea	Increases antigen-specific immunoglobulin production. Enhances killer cell cytotoxicity

- Help to reduce the behavioural changes associated with cognitive dysfunction.

- Feed a nutritionally balanced diet, aimed at the senior lifestage.

- Aim to reduce the oxidative stress by neutralizing free radicals and thus preventing extensive cellular damage.

Clinical nutrition

Proteins

The protein levels in diets aimed at animals with cognitive dysfunction need to be similar to those of senior lifestage diets. Levels tend to be around 19–20% dry matter base (DMB). This is to aid in maintaining heart and kidney health in the senior animal.

Carbohydrates

The levels of carbohydrates within the diet do need to reflect that the senior animal can be less active than a younger adult. The calorific levels of carbohydrate content can therefore be decreased. It is recommended though that the fibre content of senior diets is higher than that of adult lifestage diets. Bowel function in older dogs can be decreased, and the addition of fibre can assist in its functioning. Carbohydrate (nitrogen-free extract; NFE) levels are recommended at around 55% (DMB), and crude fibre at 4.5% (DMB).

Fats

The overall level of fats within the diet need to reflect a senior diet. The type of fats contained within the diet is important. Levels of the omega-3 fatty acids docosahexaenoic acid (DHA) and eicosapentaenoic acid (EPA) need to be increased. These fats contribute to neuronal cell membrane plasticity and health.[3] The decline in structural and functional integrity of the brain tissue correlates with the loss of DHA concentrations from the cell membranes. The brain is rich in polyunsaturated fatty acids (PUFA), especially DHA, with concentrations of PUFA directly reflecting concentrations within the diet. It has therefore been concluded that diets with increased levels of n-6 and n-3 fatty acids may help to delay or reduce the onset of neurodegenerative disorders such as cognitive dysfunction.[3]

A natural phospholipid, phosphatidylseine, has been added to some supplements designed to aid in cognitive dysfunction. The main physiological effect is to enhance and maintain the cell activities based on the functionality of the plasma membrane.

Vitamins and minerals

The levels of the vitamins and minerals that act as antioxidants are increased in diets aimed at dogs with cognitive dysfunction. This is due to the effects that the antioxidants have on protecting against free radical damage. The main antioxidants used are vitamins E and C, beta-carotene and selenium. Vitamin E is used to help neutralize free radical reactivity. Antioxidants are believed to promote recovery in neurons that are exhibiting signs of neuropathology, and therefore nutritional manipulation is believed to offer useful medication-related treatments for cognitive dysfunction. Vitamin C regenerates vitamin E, restoring its antioxidant activity. Beta-carotene reinforces vitamin E and also boosts its antioxidant capacity. Selenium in the diet aids by being a component of the antioxidant enzyme glutathione peroxidase.

The levels of other vitamins and minerals within the diet need to reflect levels required by animals at a senior lifestage.

Feeding a dog with cognitive dysfunction

Diets have been designed to encompass all of these nutritional components. The difficulty arises when the animal is suffering from another disease or disorder, and requires a diet specifically for this problem. Supplements have been designed that contain the antioxidants recommended for cognitive dysfunction. The levels of fatty acids are more

Key points

- Feed depending on the animal's body condition score (BCS) and weight. Specific cognitive dysfunction diets are aimed at animals with an ideal weight and BSC.
- Supplements can be utilized if the animal is on a specific diet for a concurrent condition.
- Cognitive dysfunction is not an inevitability of old age.

difficult to increase, but this can be achieved by using oil supplements.

As diets aimed at cognitive dysfunction are based around a senior lifestage diet, there are few side effects experienced when changing. It should be remembered that older dogs can be fussier with their diets, and transition to a new diet can be difficult. It should also be noted to owners that there is no cure for cognitive dysfunction, only aid in delaying some of the symptoms. Regular examinations at the veterinary practice should be advocated, along with medications as required.

CASE STUDY 14.1

On routine annual vaccination of her dog, an owner complained that the animal was slowing down due to old age. On further questioning it was revealed that the dog was interacting less with his family, having disturbed sleep patterns and was slightly disorientated at times. A full clinical examination was undertaken in order to rule out an underlying cause. All blood profiles proved to be normal. The dog was placed on a nutraceutical designed to aid animals displaying signs of cognitive dysfunction. The owner preferred this method because the dog was very fussy with its food and she did not want to change its diet. After supplementing the dog's diet for 6 weeks, the owner reported that the dog was starting to interact and play more, and that the sleep patterns had improved. The dog did still display some signs of disorientation.

References

1. Hayek MG, Massimino SP, Michael MS, et al. Modulation of immune response through nutraceutical interventions: implications for canine and feline health. Vet Clin Small Anim 2004; 34:229–247.
2. Frank D. Cognitive dysfunction in dogs. Hill's European Symposium on Canine Brain Ageing. 2000:22–27.
3. Youdim KA, Martin A, Joseph JA. Essential fatty acids and the brain: Possible health implications. Int J Dev Neurosci 2000; 18:383–399.

15

Musculoskeletal disorders

NUTRITION-RELATED SKELETAL DISORDERS

DEVELOPMENTAL ORTHOPAEDIC DISORDERS (DOD)

Developmental orthopaedic disorders (DOD) involve a diverse group of musculoskeletal disorders that occur in growing animals (most commonly fast-growing large- and giant-breed dogs, and horses).[1] DOD can be attributed to genetic make-up, nutritional and stress-related aetiologies. This chapter will discuss those aetiologies that are nutritionally induced. The majority of these disorders are made up of canine hip dysplasia (CHD) and dyschondroplasia (DCP) (osteochondrosis dissecans (OCD) is a similar condition, but occurs when inflammation is present and separation of a piece of articular cartilage and of the underlying bone within the joint has occurred). Other disorders under the umbrella of DOD include physitis (physeal dysplasia or epiphysitis), angular limb deformities and vertebral abnormalities (wobbler syndrome). The skeletal system is most susceptible to physical and metabolic insult during the first 12 months of life because of the heightened metabolic activity.[2] Problems associated with dietary excesses are more likely, especially in dogs fed a high-quality growth food that is further supplemented with minerals, vitamins and energy.[3] Lesions can appear in physeal or articular cartilage as disturbances of endochondral ossification.[4]

Nutritional aims are as follows:

- Feed a complete and balanced diet that does not precipitate any predisposition to DOD.

- When DOD do occur, the diet needs to limit any further damage that could be induced through poor or inadequate nutrition.

Clinical nutrition

Fats

Excessive dietary energy intake may support a growth rate that is too fast for correct skeletal development. Dietary fat is the primary contributor to excess energy intake,[2] and therefore levels should be monitored in large-breed diets, and in equine feeds, due to fats having twice the calorific density of proteins and carbohydrates. Excessive energy intake can occur easily in diets with higher fat levels. Dietary energy in excess of the animal's needs will be stored as body fat. Therefore the role of body condition score (BCS) is important, in order to monitor energy intake. Diets aimed at large and giant breed have a decreased energy density in comparison to small- and medium-breed puppy diets.

Studies conducted on equine diets demonstrated that excessive amounts of soluble carbohydrate (digestible starch) and total energy (129% of the recommendations of the National Research Council (NRC)) given to foals caused widespread lesions of DCP.[5,6] In these studies the increase in total energy was achieved by the addition of extra fats (oils) to the diet.

Protein

Diets aimed at fast-growing animals do have higher protein levels. The proteins used should be of a high quality and easily digestible. In dogs, protein excess has not shown to negatively affect calcium metabolism or skeletal development.[1] A growth diet for dogs should contain >22% protein (dry matter base; DMB) of a high biological value.[7] In equines, high-protein diets do not seem to predispose foals to DCP.[8]

Carbohydrates

The carbohydrate content of the diet needs to be balanced. Levels need to be sufficient to provide adequate calories to the animal, but not excessive to encourage excess weight gain. The type of carbohydrate within the diet is important. In cats and dogs the carbohydrate content needs to be of a highly digestible nature, especially in small breeds of dogs and kittens. In horses and rabbits the type of carbohydrate in the diet needs to reflect how they obtain calories from hindgut fermentation. Therefore the carbohydrates present need to be mainly of fibre. In kittens and small-breed puppies this level of fibre would decrease digestibility of the diet and thus, owing to limited stomach size, they would not be able to consume the quantities of calories required for growth.

Vitamins and minerals

The level of calcium within the diet is vitally important in the development of orthopaedic disorders in horses and large-breed dogs. Equally so is the ratio of calcium to phosphorus present within the diet. Excessive dietary phosphorus consistently produces lesions of DCP.[7] An excess of calcium causing hypercalcaemia will result in excess bone deposition, which will interfere with normal bone development (Table 15.1).

The role of vitamins A and D in causing skeletal problems has been well documented. Vitamin A is an essential factor in bone metabolism, especially osteoclastic activity. Deficiencies or excesses of vitamin A can lead to metabolic bone disease, but are fortunately rare due to the use of commercial balanced diets. Vitamin D's metabolites aid in the regulation of calcium metabolism and therefore skeletal development. Deficiency of vitamin D (rickets) is rare, again because of the use of commercial diets. Excessive amounts of vitamin D will lead to hypercalcaemia and hyperphosphataemia; clinical signs also include anorexia, polydipsia, polyuria, muscle weakness, generalized soft tissue mineralization and lameness.[1]

Table 15.1 Minimum daily requirements of calcium (Ca) and phosphorus (P) in growing horses

Age (months)	BW/kg	Ca (g/day)	P (g/day)
3	100	37	31
6	200	33	27
12	300	31	25
18	375	28	23
Fully grown	~ 450	23	18

Feeding animals with DOD

Puppies

The feeding of an animal with or predisposed to DOD must be done on an individual basis, as growth rates and requirements differ greatly. Physical evaluation or BCS should be performed at least every 2 weeks. Care must be given when trying to avoid developmental problems by changing to an adult maintenance diet from a puppy diet, in order to avoid excess calcium and energy levels. Maintenance foods have a lower energy density than growth diets, so the puppy must consume greater amounts of the diet to reach its energy requirements. Problems can arise if calcium levels in the two diets are similar, the puppy will end up consuming greater amounts of calcium, than if fed the growth diet.

Guidance should be given to owners that calcium supplements should not be given to growing puppies, unless prescribed by a veterinary surgeon. Owners should be made aware of the risk of developmental orthopaedic disorders, and that commercial growth diets contain all the calcium needed.

If a developmental orthopaedic disorder has occurred, then a review of the animal's diet and BCS is required. Nutrition can be used to aid in prevention of DOD, but its role once they have been acquired is limited. It should always be remembered that food manufacturers' recommendations are no more than that; reassessment of the animal over regular periods is the best method of obtaining a feeding plan and deciding how the animal should be fed.

Foals

The nutritional management of foals with lesions of DOD involves the management of any further exacerbation of the lesions and promotion of healing.[9] Three main factors have been identified in managing these foals:

1. *Dietary digestible energy levels.* The digestible energy (DE) of the diet needs to approximate to 85% of the NRC recommended levels for animals of a similar age.[9] One hundred per cent levels of crude protein, calcium, phosphorus and other nutrients are still required.

2. *Dietary copper levels.* The increase of copper in the diet may result in a subsequent increase in collagen cross-linking. Suggested levels are 30–45 mg/kg DMB.

3. *Exercise and feeding.* Foals which consume basal energy diets when exercised have an increased incidence of DOD. This can be because of extensive articular damage due to secondary trauma.[9] In cases where DOD have been diagnosed, the DE of the diet should be decreased and hand-walking exercise implemented. It should be noted that as exercise levels have been further decreased,

---

Key points

- Ensure a correct calcium to phosphorus ratio.
- Feed a controlled energy level, suitable for the individual.
- Regularly assess weight and BCS.
- Use of a growth chart is advisable in the monitoring of growth rates.

CASE STUDY 15.1

A 16-week-old German shepherd puppy was presented to a nurse-led puppy clinic. The owner reported that the pup was lame on its left foreleg, but felt that this had developed after playing on hard rough ground. After no improvement, the puppy was examined by a veterinary surgeon, and admitted for radiological surveys of both elbows and the long bones of the forelimbs. The puppy was overweight, and had a BCS of 4/5.

Lesions were evident on radiography, and medical therapy was implemented. This involved changing the puppy's diet to a large-breed diet, from a meat-based diet with calcium supplements, and the addition of nutraceuticals (glycoaminoglycans (GAGs), copper and chondroitin sulphate (CS)) designed for large-breed puppies. Exercise levels were also reduced, and the puppy was restricted to lead exercise only. The puppy's growth rate was closely monitored within nurse-led clinics, and plotted with the use of a growth chart.

so should the DE of the diet. In many cases the foal's DE requirement may only be 70–75% of NRC recommendations.

SECONDARY NUTRITIONAL HYPERPARATHYROIDISM

Secondary nutritional hyperparathyroidism or alimentary hyperparathyroidism occurs when there is a chronic insufficient calcium intake or absorption. This results in an increase in parathyroid hormone (PTH) synthesis and secretion, which in turn causes an increase in osteoclast activity, thus increasing calcitriol synthesis in the kidneys, resulting in increased calcium and phosphorus absorption from the intestine. When calcium levels do not cover the daily requirements, the skeleton acts as the only calcium reservoir.[10] Areas of calcium resorption are mainly at the endosteal surface of the diaphysis, and in the areas of cancellous bone.[10]

Incident rates are highest in young animals fed on a diet extremely low in calcium. This is frequently seen in all-meat diets. Other causes include diets that contain calcium-binding agents. Calcium levels on blood investigations will appear normal; it is therefore essential that ionized calcium levels be monitored.

Dietary therapy (calcium supplementation) is the treatment of choice. A complete balanced diet is recommended, and the calcium content needs to be up to 1.1% DMB.[10] Further supplementation can be achieved (when accelerated osteoid mineralization is required) at 50 mg Ca/kg BW, when using calcium carbonate or calcium lactate. It is important not to use calcium phosphate or bone meal as a supplement because of the phosphorus content.

ARTHRITIS

Osteoarthritis (OA) can be an exceptionally painful and crippling disease. OA or degenerative joint disease (DJD) is a chronic progressive disease characterized by pathological changes of the movable joints. Dietary manipulation can aid in the management of arthritis, and help improve the animal's mobility. Arthritis can be divided into two types:

1. degenerative types of arthritis, in which the degradation of the articular cartilage is a prominent feature
2. inflammatory arthropathies, where synovitis is the main pathological feature.

OA is the most common form of arthritis experienced in both animals and man. Management of OA includes weight control, appropriate exercise management and anti-inflammatory medications. OA is characterized by degeneration of the articular cartilage and proliferation of new bone.

Obesity is a major risk factor of OA. Weight loss must be initiated as soon as possible. Exercising and consequently weight loss can be difficult due to restrictions in mobility. When deciding on a diet for an animal with OA, it needs to meet the requirements for the animal's lifestage and body condition score.

The use of chondroprotectants and other nutraceuticals has become commonplace for cats and dogs suffering from OA (Fig. 15.1). Chondroprotective agents are reported to have three primary effects:

1. anabolic, by supporting or enhancing metabolism of chondrocytes and synoviocytes
2. catabolic, inhibiting degradative enzymes within the synovial fluid and cartilage matrix
3. antithrombolic, inhibiting the formation of thrombi in small blood vessels supplying the joint.[11]

Nutraceuticals are a category of chondroprotective agents and are defined as non-drug substances that are produced in a purified or extracted form and administered orally to provide compounds required for normal body structure and function, with the intent of improving health and well-being. Different types of nutraceuticals used in the management of OA are described below.

Fatty acids

Eicosapentaenoic acid (EPA) is the most effective n-3 polyunsaturated fatty acid (PUFA) for preventing cartilage catabolism in in vitro models. These data would suggest that supplementation of food with EPA would prove to be beneficial in slowing the rate of cartilage degradation in canine DJD (Fig. 15.2). EPA blocks the genes that produce

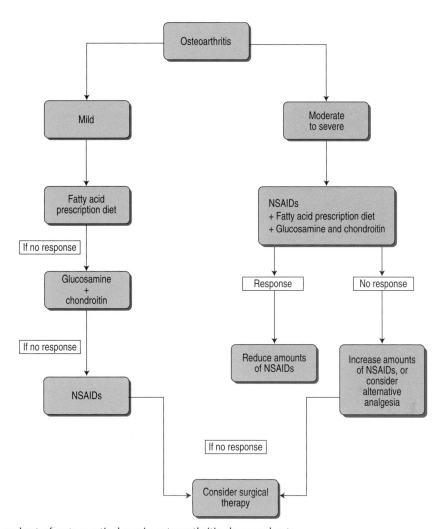

Figure 15.1 Flowchart of nutraceutical use in osteoarthritic dogs and cats.

the cartilage-destroying enzymes aggrecanase and matrix metalloproteinases (MMPs). These enzymes cause progression of the disease, even continuing after the absence of inflammation, for example if the animal is medicated with non-steroidal anti-inflammatory drugs (NSAIDs). NSAIDs stop inflammation that is caused by chondrocyte damage but do not stop degradation. The symptoms of OA are being controlled but as the damage is continuing gradual increases in medication will be required. EPA is the only omega-3 (n-3) fatty acid that is taken up by chondrocytes and remains active within the joint. EPA also helps soothe the inflammation associated with OA. Use of diets enriched with EPA have shown that the dose of

NSAIDs required to control clinical signs in dogs with OA could be reduced.[11]

The ratio of fatty acids is of great importance. High levels of omega-3 to a low level of omega-6 are required. This differs greatly from the previously used ratio of fatty acids for inflammation processes, e.g. atopy (see Ch. 10). Alpha-linolenic acid (ALA) is often supplemented in canine diets, as it is a precursor of EPA.

Glucosamine

Glucosamine supplements are the most commonly used within the OA market, and glucosamine

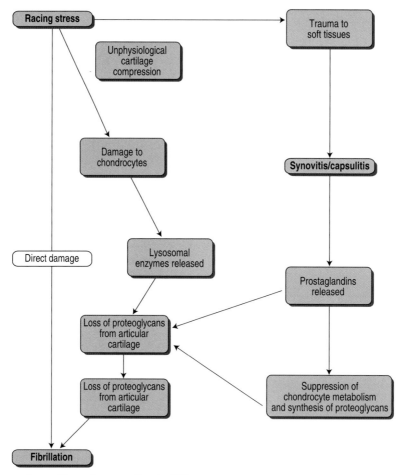

Figure 15.2 Pathways for cartilage degeneration in DJD.

hydrochloride or glucosamine sulphate are the most commonly found. Of the two, glucosamine hydrochloride will yield more glucosamine to the animal per unit weight than the sulphate form. This should be clearly explained to the owner who may wish to purchase non-veterinary products, which appear cheaper. Glucosamine is a precursor to glycoaminoglycans (GAGs), which are present in the extracellular matrix of articular cartilage. When damage occurs to chondrocytes there is a decreased ability to synthesize glucosamine; supplementing the diet stimulates the production of proteoglycans and collagen by these cells.

In traumatic degenerative joint disease (DJD), the natural balance between synthesis and degradation of cartilage shifts towards increasing degradation, resulting in loss of mucopolysaccharides. Commercially

used products are chemically similar to the mucopolysaccharides of the articular cartilage, and are concentrated into the cartilaginous tissue. Polysulphated glycoaminoglycans (PSGAGs) have been used for many years, and are routinely used as an intra-articular therapy for equine joint disease. PSGAGs have a potent ability to inhibit various lysosomal enzymes associated with proteoglycan breakdown. Some PSGAGs have been shown to be a potent inhibitor of degrading enzymes of cartilage, and stimulate the metabolism of chondrocytes and synovial cells. Experimental work with PSGAGs has indicated the prevention of further progressive degeneration within the joint and in post-surgical cases. This fact is particularly important when considering possible prophylactic schemes, especially for young animals in training.

Chondroitin sulphate

Chondroitin sulphate (CS) is another GAG present within the extracellular matrix of the articular cartilage. CS has been shown to stimulate the production of proteoglycans and collagen-like glucosamine, but can also inhibit histamine-mediated inflammation, decrease interleukin-1 production and inhibit metalloproteinases. Experimental use of oral and intramuscular CS in induced equine arthritis has shown that a decrease in articular cartilage was present, suggesting a direct anti-inflammatory effect of CS on the injury caused.[12]

Sodium hyaluronate (SH)

The mode of action of SH is unknown, but binding to the cartilage proteoglycans may slow the process of cartilage degradation, and the increase in synovial fluid viscosity may also prove to be beneficial. SH exerts an anti-inflammatory action by inhibiting the movement of granulocytes and macrophages. SH has been described as a treatment for DJD, and has been shown to be useful with synovitis, but not when obvious cartilage degeneration is present.[13]

Key points

A multimodal approach needs to be taken when considering treatments for OA. Nutritional therapy and analgesia are only two approaches; other therapies such as acupuncture, hydrotherapy, magnetic collars and modified exercise regimens should also be considered. The use of nutraceuticals in cats should be actively encouraged in the management of OA, because analgesia alternatives can be limited as there are few analgesic medications licensed for use in cats.

- Maintain optimal weight.
- Increase the use of antioxidants in order to reduce the amount of free radicals.
- Encourage the use of nutraceuticals as a supplement or as part of dietary therapy.
- Ensure mobility is maintained, and the pain levels controlled.

Postoperative uses

All surgery performed on any joint will induce some level of OA. The use of chondroprotectants has been encouraged in the postoperative period and during physical rehabilitation to accelerate and enhance recovery. Periods of immobilization should be discouraged, as reduction in synovial fluid production and proteoglycan depletion occurs due to the reduction in loading on the joint. The use of chondroprotectants aids in pain relief, so that the animal is more likely to perform physiotherapy exercises; it reduces the degradative and inflammatory enzymes which help protect the cartilage and stimulates synovial fluid, proteoglycan and collagen production to promote cartilage matrix repair.

CASE STUDY 15.2

An adult dog was presented to the veterinary practice with chronic lameness. The previous history of the dog involved a fracture to the femur and consequent osteomyelitis. The dog was anaesthetized and radiographs of both hind limbs taken. The limb with the previous history displayed severe osteoarthritis to the joint (Fig. 15.3). The dog was at its ideal weight and BCS, and no weight loss was required. The dog was placed on a diet specifically aimed at arthritic dogs, and analgesia was given. After a period of 4 days the doses of the NSAIDs were reduced, the dog displayed immediate lameness, and the NSAIDs were reintroduced. After 2 months, the NSAID dose was again reduced, the lameness did not return, and the NSAID dose was again reduced. This process was repeated until the lowest dose of NSAID that could be used was found.

EXERTIONAL RHABDOMYOLYSIS

Exertional rhabdomyolysis (ER) has many different names: azoturia, tying-up, and Monday morning disease. ER can be a severe, life-threatening condition and literally means the dissolution of striated muscle fibres following exercise.

A variety of factors are involved in the metabolic alterations of the muscle, mitochondrial function

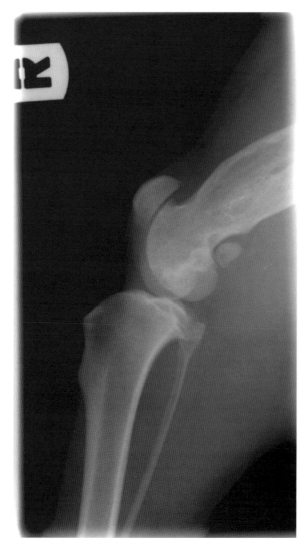

Figure 15.3 Limb of adult dog displaying severe osteoarthritis of the joint.

and electrolyte and fluid balance, making the disease pathogenesis poorly defined, and out of the scope of this text. The occurrence of recurrent ER (RER) in horses may be reduced and/or prevented by minimizing the content of cereals and sweet feed (such as molasses) in the diet.

The use of readily fermentable fibre as a feed for horses could provide an alternative to cereals in the diet. Sugar beet pulp has a high content of fermentable fibre and has been shown to be utilized in the horse, with energy content comparable to that of oats. The oral administration of electrolytes in large quantities maintains a high rate of urine flow at an alkaline pH, which prevents myoglobin precipitation in the renal tubules.[14]

Forage is, and should be, the major proportion of the daily feed intake; either pasture, hay or hay equivalents can be used. It is not preferable to feed large quantities of alfalfa or other legume-rich hays, though for horses with an increasing workload or calcium imbalance, alfalfa chaff fed in slowly increasing amounts can prove to be beneficial. The diet that is most beneficial for the sufferer will depend on each individual case. The animals' history in relationship to RER, and for what purpose it is being used, need to be taken into consideration.

Management of RER

There is no single procedure or set of protocols (including diet and management) that can guarantee against further episodes of RER. However, appropriate protocols and nutrition of susceptible animals may help to reduce the likelihood or frequency of future episodes.

1. Evaluate current management.
2. Feed forage and a maximum of 1.5–2.5 kg of sweet feed. For additional calories the use of oils is recommended.[15]
3. A regular exercise schedule should be utilized.
4. Avoid laying the horse up for more than 2 days at a time.

CASE STUDY 15.3

A 10-year-old New Forest cross pony kept at a riding stables showed clinical symptoms associated with ER. Immediate veterinary attention was sought, and the pony was kept rugged up and kept still. Analgesia was administered, and blood samples were taken to seek the severity of the problem, primarily looking at creatine kinase (CK) and aspartate aminotransferase (AST) levels. Intravenous fluids were initiated in order to ensure adequate renal perfusion and further excretion of myoglobin. The pony made an excellent recovery, and changes to its daily routine were adequately made. This involved reducing the daily ration of concentrates, and the addition of an electrolyte supplement to the diet.

LAMINITIS

Laminitis is one of the most common bilateral foot diseases in horses. The underlying cause is difficult to pinpoint, as the disease can be multifactorial. Aetiologies of laminitis include:[8]

- carbohydrate overload from a sudden grass intake (or change in pasture), after eating grain, or when supportive feeding (either TPN or PN) is initiated
- endotoxic shock (endometritis, bacterial translocation from GIT)
- allergic reactions
- poor shoeing
- lack of, or poor, foot trimming/conformation errors
- trauma from long-distance riding on hard surfaces
- weight-bearing laminitis, during box rest
- hyperadrenocorticism (Cushing's)
- exogenous glucocorticoid administration
- drinking cold water immediately after strenuous exercise
- stress of exercise in overweight animals
- excessive tube feeding of sick, aphagic horses with a high-carbohydrate–protein diet.

Insulin-resistant laminitis

It has been suggested that there is an increased level of insulin resistance in ponies prone to the development of laminitis. It has been found that laminitic ponies have lower insulin sensitivity and disposition index, and a higher acute response to glucose than normal ponies.[16] There is an existence of extreme insulin resistance and/or hyperactive insulin secretion in ponies predisposed to laminitis. The insulin resistance is likely to worsen in the face of a high consumption of starches and sugars. This has consequences of metabolic dysfunction and diseases such as laminitis and hyperlipidaemia.

Because of the many different aetiologies of laminitis there are many different treatments. This chapter will concentrate on the nutritional treatments and methods of prevention of laminitis. Restoration of the normal gut flora is required, and prevention of further endotoxin absorption. The use of a bran mash with added Epsom salts, Glauber's salts (sodium thiosulphate) or mineral oil purges can all be used to speed up the gut transit time and reduce the absorption of endotoxins. Total feed withdrawal should not occur, as this may cause hyperlipidaemia, especially in ponies. The addition of limestone to the diet when the dietary calcium to phosphorus ratio is low may have both therapeutic and prophylactic effects.

The main preventative method of inducing laminitis is the use of the correct diet. The diet that promotes the correct balance of gastrointestinal bacteria is one that contains fibre. Care should be given when changing a horse over to a diet that has higher fibre content, as sudden changes in diet can result in impaction colic.

Clinical nutrition

Carbohydrates

The main cause of laminitis is carbohydrate overload; this can be due to overeating grass or grain.[17] Essentially the flux of carbohydrate in the gut overwhelms the intestinal bacteria, resulting in abnormal fermentation. This allows a rise in the Gram-positive bacterial populations that produce lactate, notably *Streptococcus bovis*, and the proliferation of *Lactobacillus* spp. The lactate is poorly absorbed, and accumulates in the caecum and colon lowering the luminal pH, creating lactic acidosis. The normal Gram-negative bacterial population dies off, releasing endotoxins. The endotoxins enter into the bloodstream because of damage to the colonic mucosa through the bacterial changes. In horses given free access to pasture, the pH of the hindgut remains consistently around 6.4–6.7. In cases of overgrowth of undesirable bacterial populations, and lysis of desired bacterial populations, a caecal pH of below 6 is commonly noted.[17]

Starch is known to cause laminitis if sufficient quantities are consumed, but another carbohydrate, fructan, can also trigger laminitis. Fructan is a non-structural carbohydrate found in some grasses, and in certain climatic conditions (cold, bright mornings) fructan levels can increase dramatically (<50% DMB).[17] When temperatures increase, fructan accumulation is reduced as the grass grows at a better rate, using up the available sugar itself. As with cellulose, fructans cannot be metabolized by mammals, and is instead fermented by microbes in the digestive system. When large quantities of fructans are suddenly consumed, imbalances in bacterial populations within the caecum and colon occur, which can result in endotoxin release when Gram-negative bacteria die off, thus triggering the laminitis. This is why recommendations for preventing laminitis include avoiding spring grass and grazing in the morning.

Vitamins and minerals
Magnesium is known to be involved in the maintenance of normal blood sugar levels postprandially. It has also been shown to reduce the incidence of insulin resistance that has been proven to cause laminitis in native breeds, animals predisposed to laminitis and overweight/obese animals. Magnesium is also involved in the maintenance of blood circulation within the body, limbs and feet of equines. Supplementation of magnesium in the diet can be beneficial in cases of laminitis.

Key points

- Graze horses on pastures with low-fructans producing species of grass.[18]

- Turn out horses very late at night, or very early in the morning before fructan levels start increasing, bringing them off pasture by mid-morning, because fructan concentrations in the grass are at their highest at this time.

- Avoid grazing on pasture that has had a frost followed by bright sunny weather, again due to the fructans concentrations.[18]

References

1. Richardson DC, Zentek J, Hazewinkel HAW, et al. Developmental orthopaedic disease of dogs. In: Hand MS, Thatcher CD, Remillard RL, et al., eds. Small animal clinical nutrition. 4th edn. Missouri: Mark Morris Institute; 2000:505–528.
2. Richardson DC, Toll PW. Relationship of nutrition to developmental skeletal disease in young dogs. Vet Clin Nutr 1996; 3(3):6–13.
3. Kallfelz FA, Dzanis DA. An epidemic problem in pet animal practice. Vet Clin Small Anim 1989; 19(3):433–446.
4. Daemmrich K. Relationship between nutrition and bone growth in large and giant dogs. J Nutr 1991; 121:114–121.
5. Savage CJ, McCarthy RN, Jeffcott LB. Effects of dietary energy and protein on induction of dyschondroplasia in foals. Equ Vet J Suppl 1993; 16:74–79.
6. Savage CJ, McCarthy RN, Jeffcott LB. Effects of dietary phosphorus and calcium on induction of dyschondroplasia in foals. Equ Vet J Suppl 1993; 16:80–83.
7. Dzanis DA. The AFFCO dog and cat food nutrient profiles. In: Bonagura JD, ed. Current veterinary therapies XII. Philadelphia: Saunders; 1995:1418–1421.
8. Frape DF. Equine nutrition and feeding. 2nd edn. Oxford: Blackwell Science; 1998.
9. Harris PA, Frape DL, Jeffcott LB, et al. Equine nutrition and metabolic disease. In: Higgins AJ, Wright IM, eds. The equine manual. London: Saunders; 1995:123–185.
10. Hazewinkel HAW. Nutritional-related skeletal disorders. In: Ettinger SJ, Feldman EC, eds. Textbook of veterinary internal medicine, Volume 1. 6th edn. St Louis, Missouri: Elsevier Saunders; 2005:563–566.
11. Beale BS. Use of nutraceuticals and chondroprotectants in osteoarthritic dogs and cats. Vet Clin Small Anim 2004; 34(1):271–290.
12. May SA. Current research relevant to equine joint disease: animal models and other experimental systems in the investigation of equine arthritis. In: McIlwraith CW, Trotter G, eds. Joint disease in the horse. Philadelphia: Saunders; 1996.
13. McIlwraith CW, Vachon A. Review of pathogenesis and treatment of degenerative joint disease. Equ Vet J Suppl 1998; 6:3–11.

14. Valberg SJ. Tying-up in horses. Third International Conference on Feeding Horses. Applied Session. 2000:25–29.

15. Lindberg JE, Karlsson CP. Effect of partial replacement of oats with sugar beet pulp and maize oil on nutrient utilisation in horses. Equ Vet J 2001; 33(6):585–590.

16. Harris P. Nutrition studies: food for thought. Veterinary Times 2006; (11 Sept):6–8.

17. Payne R. Carbohydrate overload laminitis. Veterinary Times 2005; (10 Oct):24–27.

18. Longland AC, Cairns AJ. Fructans and their implications in the aetiology of laminitis. Proceedings of the Third International Conference on Feeding Horses. Scientific Session. April 2000:52–55.

16
Obesity

Obesity in dogs and cats

Obesity is the most prevalent form of malnutrition in pets presented to veterinary practices. Obesity is deemed to be when body fat exceeds 15–20% of bodyweight.[1] Excessive weight is an associative cause or exacerbating factor for specific orthopaedic, endocrine, cardiovascular and neoplastic disease.[2] Obesity will also make the animal less tolerant of or resilient to metabolic stress. The weight and volume of fat in the abdomen of an obese animal can exert enough pressure on the bladder to induce leakage of urine. Obesity can lead to problems associated with a reduction in grooming, especially in cats, due to an inability to reach around the abdomen (Fig. 16.1). The animal needs to change from a positive energy balance to a negative energy balance.

The aims of a nutritional management diet to promote weight loss include:

- supplying adequate nutrients, within a reduced-calorie diet
- promoting smooth weight loss, whilst maintaining lean body mass
- increasing conversion of fat to energy.

Satiation is related to the rate of food consumption (an animal can overeat before realizing that it is satiated), and food constituents (protein is more satiating than carbohydrates) and the animal's sense of fullness. These three factors should be used in the construction of a dietary plan for obesity control. Nutritional management only comprises part of a weight loss management programme; the animal's exercise levels and lifestyle also need to be considered.

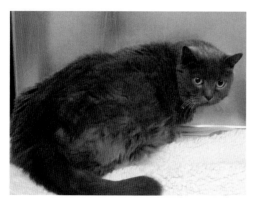

Figure 16.1   Obesity can lead to reduced grooming.

Clinical nutrition

Protein

Diets with high protein levels can be classed as low-energy diets, in comparison to those that are high in carbohydrates (Table 16.1). These diets can be advantageous as they conserve lean body mass whilst being efficient in inducing weight loss in cats. Values stated as kcal per gram are usually of metabolized energy not net energy. By using the net energy fraction, calorie differences are greater, highlighting the advantages of using a high-protein diet in cats.[3]

Carbohydrates

The role of carbohydrates in an obesity diet can be vital. The method by which obesity diets work can

be in altering the levels of non-fermentable fibres. The role of the fibre is to achieve the sensation of satiety in the animal while it is receiving a reduced proportion of calories within its diet. In some high-fibre obesity diets this can mean that only 60% of the animal's daily calorific requirement is obtained from the diet. The other 40% is obtained from utilization of the animal's bodily fat reserves. High-fibre diets in cats may affect object play, and therefore reduce calorie expenditure.

This high level of fibre can have its disadvantages, which should be clearly explained to the owner if the weight loss plan is to be successful. These disadvantages include the increase in faecal output and possibly flatulence.

Fats

The fat level in an obesity diet does need to be restricted, in order to control calorific intake. The diet should, however, contain necessary levels of the essential fatty acids (EFA). Some obesity diets aid in weight loss by only providing the animal with ~60–70% of its daily energy requirements. The required energy shortfall is met by utilization of the animal's bodily fat stores.

Vitamins and minerals

The oxidative cell damage caused by free radicals is higher in obese animals. It is therefore recommended that the diet be supplemented with antioxidants. If comparing diets on a calorific value,

Table 16.1   Calorific value of nutrients

	1 g carbohydrate	1 g protein	1 g fat
GE	4.2 kcal	5.4 kcal	9.4 kcal
GE → DE			
True energy value	3.7 kcal	4.8 kcal	8.5 kcal
% of GE	88%	89%	90%
DE → ME			
True energy value	3.5 kcal	3.5 kcal	8.5 kcal
% of GE	83%	65%	90%
ME → NE			
True energy value	3.2 kcal	2.2 kcal	8.2 kcal
% of GE	76%	41%	87%

GE, gross energy; DE, digestible energy; ME, metabolizable energy; NE, net energy.

vitamin and mineral levels in these diets will seem higher. This is due to the low-calorie nature of the diet. When comparing nutrient levels in these diets it is advisable to use other quantitative values. The typical vitamin and mineral values should be sufficient for the lifestage of that particular individual.

L-Carnitine

L-Carnitine (beta-hydroxy-γ-trimethylaminobutyric acid) is a small water-soluble vitamin-like molecule.[4] L-Carnitine is concentrated in mammalian cardiac and skeletal muscle by an active membrane transport mechanism. It has been shown to increase body fat loss and prevent loss of muscle mass,[5] and can also protect cats from hepatic lipid accumulation during calorie restriction.[6] Most obesity diets contain supplemented levels of L-carnitine.

Supplements

Liquid supplements can be used in combination with dietary and exercise management. The supplement mitratapide is a potent microsomal triglycerides transfer protein (MTP) inhibitor. The effect is to block the uptake of dietary lipids, and to enhance satiety. These supplements have some use in animals that have difficulty losing weight because of owner non-compliance, or in dogs that refuse specific diets aimed at obesity control. Additional supplementing with vitamins and minerals is not required, even though the absorption of the fat-soluble vitamins is reduced in the process. This is due to the large levels of fat-soluble vitamins present in the adipose tissue. The dog should, however, receive a complete balanced diet.

It is vital in these cases that specific dietary and exercise regimens are established whilst using mitratapide supplements, as they are initially used only for an 8-week period. If the dog's target weight has not been reached within this 8-week period, weight loss needs to be achieved through management regimens. Mitratapide supplements can be re-administered, but a minimum of 1 month should be left before re-prescribing.

Feeding an obesity diet

Weight reduction programmes initiated within the veterinary practice do tend to be more successful, mainly due to close monitoring and the support offered. Programmes include three important stages:

a feeding plan, based on the amount of excess fat to be lost and what is currently being fed; an exercise plan, based on mobility allowances and the owner's lifestyle and job commitments; and a recheck plan. Reduced calorie intake alone will not substantially reduce weight. For the weight reduction to be a success, all three stages of the programme must be completed. Stage 3, the recheck plan, will depend on the case history, success of weight loss and the practice policy.

In order to correctly design a feeding plan, the ideal bodyweight of the animal needs to be obtained. An ideal or optimal bodyweight should be calculated by examining the animal. Using body condition score (BCS) is the preferred way to assess the animal as it takes into account the animal's frame size independent of its weight. The animal's coat can also prove to be quite deceptive in obscuring an underweight or overweight animal. Dogs and cats that have an optimal body condition score have normal body contours; the bony prominences can be palpated readily under the skin surfaces. Once an ideal bodyweight has been calculated, the amount of weight to be lost is known. Some therapeutic or prescription diets require the animal to be fed a set amount depending on the ideal bodyweight and adjustment thereafter from this quantity in 10% increments. Evaluating the animal's diet, and removing all titbits and snacks will aid in an initial loss of weight. This strategy will give limited weight loss in most animals. Reduction in quantities of a maintenance diet can lead to deficiencies in important nutrients, and should be avoided.

The disadvantages of using high-fibre diets should be explained to the owners. Increases in defecation and faecal output if not explained can cause the owner to cease feeding the diet. Encouraging the owner to feed the last daily diet earlier, and giving the animal either more access to the litter tray or an increased ability to go outside, will eliminate any problems. The correct approach is to feed 60% of the maintenance rate for the animal's bodyweight. Fat will then be utilized to provide the shortfall supply.

Once the ideal weight has been achieved, maintaining this optimal weight can be difficult, and even more frequent weight check-ups may be required. Owner encouragement is still recommended to keep up established exercise regimens and positive feeding habits, as lost weight can easily be regained. Dogs and cats experience a 'rebound' effect following weight loss if fed an uncontrolled diet.[7] Selection of a new diet once the optimal weight has been achieved can be difficult, and can vary from animal to animal. Some will maintain the optimal weight well on a light lifestage diet combined with an exercise programme. Others will require a modified amount of the obesity diet or a transitional therapeutic weight control diet.

The length of time required to reach optimal weight depends on the individual patient. It can be calculated by:

$$\frac{\text{Initial BW (g)} - \text{Target BW (g)}}{\text{Weekly weight loss (g)}} = \text{Time to reach target BW (weeks)}$$

The weekly weight loss can differ from week to week, especially in cats whose activity levels can vary greatly, especially depending on the weather. In multicat households there is often one fat cat and one or more lean cats. Play and activity feeding should be emphasized. Tunnels or small holes for feeding access that the fat cat cannot get through can be utilized for the leaner cats.

Obesity in equines

Obesity in horses has been associated with an increased risk of laminitis, hyperlipidaemia, heat intolerance, and insulin insensitivity, as well as an increased risk of developmental orthopaedic disorders (DOD). Most cases of obesity are linked to an energy imbalance. Correction of the imbalance is to increase energy expenditure, through exercise, and to reduce food intake, whether concentrates or grass. Obese horses when sick can be poorly tolerant of even short periods of anorexia. Hypertriglyceridaemia (>50 mg/dl) and/or recognition of cloudy, opaque plasma or serum suggest hyperlipidaemia, and the risk of development of liver dysfunction from hepatic lipidosis.[8]

Obesity in rabbits

Obesity in rabbits is starting to become more common. This is mainly due to the inappropriate diets that rabbits are being fed, and to lack of exercise. Obesity and poor diet can be a major causative factor for the development of myiasis. In many cases the rabbit is too large to practice caecotrophy, and the sticky caecotrophs attract flies. Careful dietary modification needs to occur in these cases. Any dramatic changes in diet, even to a more nutritious

Key points

- Communication to the owner about feeding regimens is vital if weight loss is to occur.
- Consideration of all factors, e.g. exercise regimen, number of pets in the household, etc., must be made if successful weight loss is to happen.

CASE STUDY 16.1

A large 9.2-kg cat was initially presented to obesity clinics for weight loss. The cat was placed onto an appropriate weight-loss programme. Little success was gained from the weight-loss programme despite efforts from the owner and 10% decreases in feeding quantities. The cat was being weighed on a monthly basis because of owner commitments; on one visit the cat had dramatically dropped from just under 9 kg down to 8.2 kg. From a weight point of view this was excellent, but it did not follow the pattern of weight loss that the cat had experienced, i.e. very little at all. After explaining this to the veterinary surgeon, it was decided to monitor the cat, and reweigh in 2 weeks, with the cat remaining on the same quantity of diet. Within the next week the cat developed signs of lethargy, subnormal temperature, inappetence and dehydration. In-house blood testing showed various elevations in blood biochemistry (Table 16.2).

This case highlights the importance of careful monitoring of obesity cases. The weight loss in this case could have been attributed to what was suspected to be chronic renal failure. Unfortunately the cat did not respond to intensive fluid therapy and medications, and was euthanized at the owner's request.

Table 16.2 Biochemistry parameters of cat in Case Study 16.2

Biochemistry	Level
Amylase	1581 U/l
Urea	>46.41 mmol/l
Choline	11.11 mmol/l
Creatinine	879 µmol/l
Glucose	10.42 mmol/l
Phosphorus	>5.19 mmol/l
Total bilirubin	49 µmol/l
Total protein	96 g/l
Globulin	66 g/l

CASE STUDY 16.2

A Welsh springer spaniel was referred to weight clinics after gaining 6 kg after being placed on phenobarbital in order to control seizures. This medication does increase appetite in some cases, and had been the causal factor in this case. The patient was unstable, and the veterinary surgeon also started to administer potassium bromide as a conjunctive therapy. In these cases high-fibre obesity diets are usually utilized. Care needs to be taken that the high fibre content does not interfere with the drugs, by binding them up.

The dog was placed onto the high-fibre obesity diet, and the owner was advised that the tablets should not be administered at the same time as feeding.

one, will have damaging effects. Dietary changes must occur every slowly; starvation is not an option in rabbits, owing to the chance of inducing hepatic lipidosis. An ideal diet must be low in calories and high in fibre; in many of these cases the removal of all inappropriate foodstuffs and an increase in roughage (grass and hay) and vegetables is all that is required. Low-calorie pelleted diets are available on the market, but these are no substitute for a good all-round balanced diet, combined with exercise.

References

1. Debraekaleer J. Obesity in cats and dogs. Veterinary Times 2004; (22 March):14.
2. Biourge V. Obesity, a major risk factor for diabetes in cats. Royal Canin's guide to feline obesity. Royal Canin Publications; 2001:10–13.
3. Martin L. The principle of high-protein diets and net energy. Royal Canin's guide to feline obesity. Royal Canin Publications; 2001:6–9.
4. Pion PD. Traditional and non-traditional effective and noneffective therapies for cardiac disease in dogs and cats. Vet Clin Small Anim 2004; 34:187–216.
5. Armstrong PJ, Hardie EM, Cullen JM. L-Carnitine reduces hepatic fat accumulation during rapid weight reduction in cats. Proceedings of the 10th Veterinary Medical Forum. 1992:810.
6. Gross KL, Wedekind KJ, Kirk CA. Effect of dietary carnitine or chromium on weight loss and body composition of obese dogs. Proceedings of the American Society of Animal Science. 1998. Online. Available: http://www.asas.org/jas/symposia/proceedings.
7. LaFlamme DP, Kuhlman G. The effect of weight loss on subsequent weight maintenance in dogs. J Vet Intern Med 1993; 7(134).
8. Goer RJ. Nutritional support of the sick adult horse. In: Pagan JD, Geor RJ, eds. Advances in equine nutrition II. Kentucky: Kentucky Equine Research; 2000:403–417.

17
Perioperative feeding

Cats and dogs

Preoperative feeding

Preoperative fasting of patients being administered a general anaesthetic or heavy sedation is widely established in veterinary practice. This is due to the reduction in risk of vomiting, regurgitation and possible aspiration of gastric contents during or while recovering from anaesthesia.[1] If the animal has consumed solids during the previous 4 hours, or clear fluids during the previous 2 hours, the general anaesthetic should be delayed if possible, in order to allow the stomach to empty.[2] Inadequate fasting can cause severe complications and must be avoided. The use of pre-anaesthetic blood work-ups should be recommended for all patients, and can highlight any underlying diseases, assess hydration levels, and identify any electrolyte imbalances. The hydration levels of the animal must be assessed before every anaesthetic or sedation performed.

The length of time that patients should fast is controversial, and is dependent on the length of time it takes food to pass through the stomach, the nature of the meal consumed, and the fact that the stomach is never truly empty.[3] Carbohydrates leave the stomach more rapidly than protein, while fat is the slowest to leave.[2] It has been proposed in human nursing that a prolonged fasting time could cause nausea preoperatively, which might then persist into the postoperative recovery period.[4] Food-fasting for more than 6 hours can reduce the body's ability to cope with stressors such as blood loss or infection.[5] Older, sick or debilitated patients are at greater risk of dehydration, malnutrition and electrolyte imbalances; fasting times in these patients should not be excessive, with fluids being removed only 2 hours prior to induction of anaesthesia. The nature of the procedure also needs to be taken into account. The presence of faecal matter in the colon when performing diagnostic imagery can cause difficulties. Enemas can be used to remove residual faeces and clean the rectum. In these cases a longer period of withheld solids is necessary, but water should not be withheld until at least 2 hours pre-induction.

Postoperative feeding

After any surgery, supportive nutrition is required. Surgery, even minor surgery, has an illness factor of 1.25 × resting energy requirements (RER). Nutrient requirements are increased in order for repair to occur. In the immediate postoperative period, the diet needs to be highly digestible, palatable and provide adequate calories. Once the animal has recovered sufficiently, fresh water should be made available, then food should be offered. It should be noted that due to the period of preoperative starvation the patient will be hungry. As many animals, especially cats, obtain the majority of their daily water requirement from their diet, provision of a moist postoperative diet is advantageous. Offering food before the animal has sufficiently recovered can be dangerous.

When surgery involves the gastrointestinal tract, nutritional support still needs to be initiated. In cases of surgery that contraindicate feeding orally (e.g. oral surgery), enteral nutritional support via tube feeding should be administered. In the past any animal that underwent gastrointestinal surgery was starved for 24 hours postoperatively. This practice has been shown to be detrimental to the animal's health and rate of recovery from the initial problem.

When prolonged starvation occurs, the gastrointestinal muscle atrophies and predisposes to bacterial translocation. This occurs as a result of the intestinal mucosa losing its integrity, and allows the normal enteric flora to pass into the bloodstream and become systemic. Bacteraemia and septicaemia can result. This can occur when the animal is placed on parenteral feeding, although contamination of the central venous line site can also cause bacteraemia and septicaemia. Very small amounts of a highly digestible food should be given by mouth, as the consequence of bacterial translocation outweighs that of giving the food.[1]

The nutrients within the intestinal lumen not only provide the animal with nourishment, but also the enterocytes. The enterocytes gain nutrients from the lumen, rather than from the vascular system. Decreases in enterocyte populations can cause otherwise inhibited potentially pathogenic bacterial populations to increase. Nutrients within the intestinal lumen also aid in immunity, stimulate the brush order activity and stimulate development of villi.[2] Glutamine (one of the amino acids utilized in gut development) that is administered intravenously cannot be utilized by the small intestine, and this is where the breakdown occurs.

When surgery is within the gastrointestinal tract and sutures or staples are placed, common feeding principles were to starve the animal for 24 hours. Questions have been raised over how the gut can heal if there are no nutrients present in order to stimulate villus development; and clearly the gut takes longer than 24 hours to 'heal' postoperatively. Once sutures have been placed, they only lose integrity; they do not gain it. Feeding when the sutures are at their structural strongest is preferred.

The ideal diet postoperatively is one that is highly digestible, low in fibre, low in fat and has a low residue. Electrolyte levels need to be balanced in order to aid in any correction of losses through vomiting or diarrhoea.

Key points

Preoperative

- Patients should only be starved of solids for 4–6 hours; this also includes milk.
- Fasting times should be individualized taking into account the patient's age and nutritional status, and also the procedure being undertaken.

Postoperative

- All patients require some form of nutrition as soon as possible postoperatively. If enteral methods are not possible, parenteral methods should be commenced.
- Any form of surgery places an increased nutrient demand on the body.
- When able to consume solids, a highly digestible, low-fat diet should be used.

Rabbits

Preoperative feeding

Stabilization of the animal prior to any surgery is vital, but unfortunately undervalued. Many rabbits presented to the veterinary practice due to inappetence require dentistry. Removal of any simple, quickly solved problems (i.e. burring of teeth) and the use of analgesia can make the animal more comfortable for a couple of days whilst supportive nutrition is administered. This can be through nasogastric tubes or syringe feeding. Any more complicated dental work can then be performed when the animal is more stable.

The animal's hydration status should always be assessed. The tenting of skin in rabbits is an indication of poor hydration levels. Where animals have been obtaining a large proportion of their daily water content from their diet, and now have a reduced food intake or anorexia, measures must be made to actively increase water consumption (Appendix 4). It is always advisable for a blood work-up to be performed prior to surgery in order to highlight any potential problems.

Vomiting is not possible in these animals, but regurgitation is. Removal of food 1–2 hours preoperatively is recommended.

Postoperative feeding

Rabbits, unless contraindicated, should be allowed to eat as soon as it is safe. Rabbits should be allowed to recover from anaesthetics on a bed of clean, dust-free hay. Many rabbits will start to nibble at hay or grass even before they are willing to stand. Supportive feeding methods should be utilized in these animals if inappetence occurs. Rabbits should not be discharged postoperatively until eating has been established, and normal faeces are being produced.

Equines

Preoperative feeding

The optimal length of preoperative starvation is 12–24 hours; the main aim of this is to reduce gut fill. However, the reduction in the GIT volume can facilitate anaesthesia, especially respiratory function, and aid in moving the animal. Starvation for periods longer than this can delay wound healing and depress the immune function.

Consideration should be given to the maintenance diet of horses that are going to be hospitalized for a period of time. High levels of concentrates are not appropriate for horses that are going to be hospitalized for more than a day or two.[6] Care should be taken that no sudden dramatic changes are made to the diet, as GIT disturbances can occur.

Postoperative feeding

Postoperative feeding depends on the nature of the surgery that has been undertaken. Where surgery does not affect the GIT, hay should be made available to the horse as soon as completely recovered from anaesthesia. Any concentrate feeds should be reintroduced gradually. Surgery that affects the GIT deserves special consideration, with the overall success dependent not only on the surgery, but mainly on the postoperative nutrition. In many practices, water is not often first choice following surgery as it tends to sit in the stomach. Most often, grass is offered for 2–3 minutes two or three times daily, gradually increasing; then small handfuls of soaked hay, and water; then moving up to bran mashes. Hydration levels can be maintained through the use of intravenous fluid therapy. Many horses will take roughly 4–5 days before returning to normal rations.

Colic

The protocol for postoperative nutrition after surgical intervention is largely dependent on the surgery undertaken. All types of colic surgery predispose to diarrhoea,[7] the incidence following large colon surgery being higher than after surgery to the small intestine. Recommendations are to feed grass hay to horses following large colon surgery for 1–2 weeks.[6] An early introduction of soft grass hay in all postoperative cases will stimulate GI motility, and provide a source of potassium. Hypokalaemia is a common intraoperative and postoperative problem, often compounded by the absence of food.[6] Post-surgical access to grass is always the most beneficial to the horse. Recovering horses do need a higher nutrient and water intake, similarly to other species, in order for recovery to occur.

As in small animal surgery there are conflicting views surrounding the feeding of animals that have undergone GIT surgery. Horses have large metabolic reserves compared to other companion animals, but food deprivation for longer periods of time can still induce bacterial translocation, as described in postoperative feeding for cats and dogs. Soft mashes or gruels from ground feeds or grass will pass through the small intestine readily, reduce distension at the site of anastomosis and reduce physical factors contributing towards the breakdown of the anastomosis.[6] Bran mashes are commonly used, but bran does act as a bulk laxative and can have a low palatability.

When resections have occurred, the ongoing diet of the animal needs to be addressed. Depending on the type of resection, the animal's digestive abilities will be impaired. Resection of the small intestine can lead to malabsorptions, weight loss, lethargy and diarrhoea.[8] Once a horse has undergone surgery for colic it is more likely for colic to recur.[6] Certain types of roughage seem to predispose these animals to repeated episodes. These types of roughage tend to have high fibre content and should be avoided. In many cases horses can be starved 48 hours postoperatively for small intestinal resections, but less than 24 hours for large colon torsions.

Oesophageal surgery

Nutritional management of animals that have undergone oesophageal surgery needs to be specialized for roughly 2 months. The feeding of a traditional hay–grain diet will have severe detrimental effects. The two major nutritional concerns with oesophageal problems are electrolyte imbalance and wound healing.[6] The feeding of a slurry or liquid diet via a feeding tube must be instigated. This can be a nasogastric or oesophageal tube until the mucosal lesion is healed. The horse should be left on a soft diet for a minimum of 30–45 days after surgery.[6]

Rectal surgery

Nutritional management of horses that have undergone rectal surgery requires a laxative diet in order to reduce the pressure on the suture lines. Commonly used diets include fresh grass, and complete diets based on finely ground alfalfa. Grinding alfalfa decreases passage time and increases faecal water content.[9]

References

1. Seymour S. Preoperative fluid restriction: hospital policy and clinical practice. Brit J Nursing 2000; 9(14):925–930.
2. Webb K. What are the pitfalls of preoperative fasting? Nursing Times 2003; 99(50):41–45.
3. Hillier M. Exploring the evidence around preoperative fasting practices. Nursing Times 2006; 10(28):36–38.
4. Smith A. Shorter preoperative fluid fasts reduce postoperative emesis. Br Med J 1997; 314:1092–1486.
5. Hall E. Gastrointestinal problems. In: Kelly N, Wills J, eds. BSAVA manual of companion animal nutrition and feeding. Gloucester: BSAVA Publications; 1996:144–152.
6. Naylor JM. What to feed pre- and post surgery. Proceedings of the BEVA Specialist Days on Behaviour and Nutrition; 1999:87–90.
7. Hird DW, Casebolt DB, Carter JD, et al. Risk factors for salmonellosis in hospitalised horses. J Am Vet Res 1986; 188:173–177.
8. Tate LP Jr, Ralston SL, Koch CM, et al. Effects of extensive resection of the small intestine in the pony. Am J Vet Res 1983; 44:1187–1191.
9. Hintz HF, Loy RG. Effect of pelleting on the nutritive value of horse rations. J Anim Sci 1966; 25:1059–1062.

18
Urinary system

Chapter contents

RENAL FAILURE

In all animals, clinical symptoms of renal dysfunction are not evident until 65–75% of renal tissue has been destroyed (Table 18.1). Nutritional management can affect many consequences of renal failure, and is the cornerstone of management. Chronic renal failure (CRF) has many physiological effects; these include the decreased ability to excrete nitrogenous waste (and consequently the development of azotaemia), sodium and phosphorus, and an increased loss of potassium. Other clinical symptoms include systemic hypertension, secondary hyperparathyroidism and non-regenerative anaemia.[1] The aim therefore is:

- to aid in the preservation of the remaining renal tissue
- to reduce accumulation of nitrogenous waste in the bloodstream (azotaemia) by minimizing protein precursors for urea
- to correct fluid, electrolyte and acid–base balance
- to provide adequate calories to prevent further catabolism or malnutrition.

Clinical nutrition
Water

Renal disease causes a progressive decline in urine concentrating capacity. Dehydration, volume depletion, renal hypoperfusion and dietary salt intake stimulate urine concentration, though avoiding dehydration and renal hypoperfusion reduces the work of concentrating the urine and helps to maintain intrarenal protective mechanisms. Patients with CRF must have unlimited access to fresh water

Table 18.1 Signs of CRF in line with the quantity of nephrons destroyed

Approximate percentage of nephrons destroyed	Signs of renal failure
66%	Reduced capacity for urine concentration, lower specific density of urine
75%	Azotaemia. Increased serum urea and creatinine
85%	Increased serum phosphorus

and free choice consumption. This can be exceptionally important in cats, which have fastidious drinking habits.

Increasing water consumption can be achieved in a number of different ways, for example by feeding a moist diet rather than a dry diet, and by increasing the availability of water by placing more bowls around the house and in the garden. Allowing water to stand for a period of time prior to being offered to some animals can be beneficial. This allows the chlorine in the water to evaporate off, which some animals prefer. Further details are provided in Appendix 4.

Protein
The majority of veterinary diets for dogs are in two 'phases', indicated for the different stages of CRF. This staged management system is recommended in dogs, as early cases can benefit from phosphorus restriction, whilst maintaining a protein intake level equal to an adult maintenance level. Early cases are defined as those that are azotaemic and not uraemic, and make up 18–20% of dogs suffering from CRF.[2]

For dogs with uraemia at presentation, the diet needs to have a lower protein level. This will help to reduce the protein catabolites that are produced. The protein that is present in these diets needs to be of a high biological value to minimize the risk of essential amino acid deficiency. If protein is too restricted in both cats and dogs with CRF, hypoalbuminaemia, anaemia and metabolic acidosis can occur. It is, therefore, important to gain the correct balance of protein levels. If protein levels are too high, protein can act as a source of calories through deamination in the liver, and the nitrogenous waste products will then exacerbate the azotaemia.

Previous studies have implicated dietary protein as a direct possible cause of CRF, or a cause of decreased function in already dysfunctioning kidneys.[3] The majority of these studies were conducted with rats. Subsequently, studies have identified that the dog (and possibly cat, horse and rabbit) are different from the rat in response to dietary protein.[3]

Proteinuria of glomerular origin was traditionally considered to be a consequence of damage to the glomerular barrier.[4] But some studies have discovered that proteinuria observed in association with an increased protein intake may be related to haemodynamic alteration and physiological changes in glomerular permeability selectivity, rather than damage to the glomerular filtration barrier.[4] An increase in protein excretion in urine is attributed to the passage of time (wear and tear) rather than protein and phosphorus levels,[4] and underlines that urinalysis is a valuable and often under-utilized diagnostic tool in detecting CRF and its severity.

The level of protein restriction in cats, however, is important. Veterinary diets designed for renal management in cats do not have staged protein restriction levels. This is because cats cannot reduce their enzyme activity in the liver. These enzymes are involved in protein catabolism, and if the dietary protein level is greatly restricted, then protein malnutrition can occur. As with dogs, the protein level should be adequate for the animal's needs, but not too high so that excess is used as an energy source.

Vitamins and minerals
Sodium levels in renal diets are reduced. This is because of the reduction in the number of viable nephrons within the kidneys. As serum sodium levels remain the same, this means that each nephron has an increased load delivery. This, in turn, will create hypertension, as the blood pressure rises. Hence, blood pressure monitoring in animals with renal dysfunction is recommended. Sodium levels should, however, not be too restricted, as this can result in a reduced capacity to reabsorb bicarbonate. This will contribute towards metabolic acidosis. If sodium intake is rapidly reduced, dehydration and volume contraction may occur. A gradual change

in diet is recommended when changing to a salt-restricted diet, because of this and a perceived decrease in palatability. Sodium levels in renal diets are recommended at 0.3% (dry matter base; DMB) in cats and 0.2% (DMB) in dogs.[1]

Phosphorus is absorbed from the GIT, and primarily excreted by the kidneys. A restriction in dietary phosphorus has been shown to slow the progression of renal failure in cats and dogs. Hyperphosphataemia is a common finding in patients with chronic renal failure, and occurs when the glomerular filtration rate (GFR) falls below 20% of the norm. Consequently, this results in reduced renal phosphate excretion, and hence raised serum levels. This can result in renal mineralization, secondary hyperparathyroidism, thereby exacerbating renal damage, and aid in the development of hyperlipidaemia. If dietary means alone do not reduce serum phosphorus levels, then oral phosphorus-binding agents can be used. It has been shown that cats that have low phosphate levels within their diets live almost two and a half times longer that cats that are fed normal diets.[5]

Potassium deficiency has been identified in cats with CRF.[6] Hypokalaemia also impairs protein synthesis, promotes weight loss, a poor hair coat and contributes to polyuria by decreasing the renal responsiveness to antidiuretic hormone (ADH).[7]

Metabolic acidosis should be prevented, as it may be associated with increased ammoniagenesis and the progression of renal disease. If acidosis is present, an alkalinizing agent should be added to the diet. As sodium bicarbonate will increase sodium levels, either potassium or calcium carbonate can be used. Some veterinary diets adjust the levels of potassium in order to help prevent acidosis, but as each case is different, monitoring of the acid–base balance is recommended.

It is important to remember that with any disease or disorder that shows the clinical symptoms of polydipsia (PD) and polyuria (PU), water-soluble vitamins can be lost. Water-soluble vitamin deficiency can further contribute to anorexia, as even higher demands are placed on these vitamins, as the body tries to recuperate. Further supplementation with water-soluble vitamins is often not required as commercially available veterinary diets contain additional quantities of these vitamins.

Fats

As discussed earlier, the renal patient needs to gain calories from a non-protein source. This can be from fats (lipids) and carbohydrates. The addition of fats to the diet is beneficial, as fat offers twice the energy per gram as carbohydrate and aids in palatability. The use of fatty acids has also been shown to decrease inflammation in the kidney, lowers hypertension and preserves renal function; therefore veterinary diets are supplemented with omega fatty acids or polyunsaturated fatty acids, especially EPA and arachidonic acid.[6] Omega-6 fatty acids appear to be detrimental in dogs with naturally occurring renal disease by acutely increasing glomerular filtration rate.

Carbohydrates

Most manufacturers of veterinary diets do not raise the importance of dietary fibre in the management of renal disease. The animal itself cannot digest soluble fibre in the diet, but the microbes within the intestine can. Soluble fibre is fermented into short-chain fatty acids (SCFA) or volatile fatty acids (VFA). These products are an important energy source for the intestinal cells and can increase blood flow to the intestine.

Nitrogenous waste products in the blood are presented to the intestinal lumen where urease, an enzyme produced by intestinal bacteria, hydrolyses the urea into ammonia and carbon dioxide. The ammonia is then utilized by the intestinal bacteria. This process means that nitrogenous waste products are excreted in faecal matter, rather than in urine by the kidneys. Dietary fibre may also be beneficial for improving gastrointestinal motility in dogs with renal failure. Colonic transit times can be decreased in moderate renal disease as it alters duodenojejunal motility.

Supplements

Supplements that can be used in cases of chronic renal diseases are designed to help reduce the phosphate levels in the diet. Phosphate binders that can be used include calcium carbonate, which can reduce the apparent digestibility of phosphorus by more than twice what it would be when fed a standard diet.

Chitosan (a derivative of chitin) has also been used in supplements for animals suffering from chronic renal failure. Chitosan acts as an absorbent in the intestines, and thus lowers the absorption of certain substances including phosphates and some uraemic toxins.

Feeding a renal diet

Objectively, the role of these veterinary diets is to help reduce azotaemia, and hyperphosphataemia, and also to control secondary hyperparathyroidism – ultimately improving both the clinical and bio-chemical status of the animal. But a reduced dietary intake has often been blamed on the palatability of the diet. The effect of uraemia on the senses of taste and smell and the development of food aversions can all contribute towards inappetence. Changing any animal from a high-salt, high-protein diet to a commercial renal diet can be very difficult. Changing via a transitional intermediate diet over a more prolonged period of time can be beneficial in these animals. Also refer to feeding a low-salt diet on page 69.

The monitoring of animals with CRF is very important and is under-utilized. Regular monitoring to ensure dietary and medical management remains optimal for each individual animal but is vital for long-term successful management. Compliance from the owner can also be improved with this extra support from the veterinary practice. The processes of the disease should be monitored; this will include laboratory evaluation, blood pressure monitoring, full clinical history, physical examination, body-weight and body condition score (BCS). History should also be taken on the amount of food and water being consumed. Owners do find it difficult to differentiate between time spent at the food or water bowl and actual amount consumed. Careful questioning might have to be adopted.

When initiating an animal onto a renal diet, a gradual transitional period is required. Gradual changes through a range of diets from adult to senior to early renal can be beneficial for the more stubborn of animals, but can also prove of use with owners with preconceptions of changing an animal from a supermarket high-salt brand to one of restricted salt and reduced protein levels. Because of the decrease of protein in the diet, there is a relative increase in the fat and carbohydrate levels, resulting in an increase in calorific value and probable palatability due to the fat content. The increase in fat content can also cause digestive upsets such as diarrhoea. If the dietary transition has been obtained over a gradual period of time then this side effect is not common. If, however, the diarrhoea persists as soon as the renal diet makes up a certain percentage of the diet, addition of a high-fibre diet can resolve the problem. The quantity of food fed may need to be adjusted as the energy density of the new food may differ from the original.

Supporting the owner during the transition period of diet change is important, as the majority of affected animals are older, fastidious cats, some of which have very precise food preferences. A list of foods that should not be added to any commercial clinical diet can prove to be useful for the owner.

Feeding habits of animals suffering from renal failure will alter, especially if the animal is uraemic and suffering from anorexia and nausea. Small frequent meals can prove beneficial, as does providing the right feeding location and presentation. Food aversions can be a large problem with these animals, and if a clinical diet is flatly refused phosphate binders can prove to be useful.

CRF in equines

Azotaemia and hypercalcaemia are both the result of inadequate renal excretion in the horse, and are clinical symptoms of CRF. Dietary management of CRF includes avoiding foodstuffs high in protein (legumes, soya beans), phosphorus (wheat bran), and calcium (wheat bran, beet pulp, legumes and supplements). Monitoring blood protein levels is required, as hypoproteinaemia can develop. If the blood test shows hypoproteinaemia, increase in the quantity of protein within the diet is needed. Hypercalcaemia as a result of renal disease is unusual in dogs and cats, because calcium is more closely regulated than phosphorus, but in the horse it can be a problem. It is recommended that 8–10% of the diet should consist of protein, and only 0.25% as phosphorus. Calcium levels should be < 0.45% DMB.

These animals may require an increase in energy density of the diet. This can be achieved by the addition of fats (oils) to the diet. The use of omega-3 PUFA is advocated due to the anti-inflammatory effects.

CRF in rabbits

Symptomatic treatment of clinical signs is the only treatment available for CRF, the same as with other species. As in equines, dietary calcium restriction is beneficial, due to an impaired renal excretion of calcium.[7] Foods such as fresh grass, carrots, apples and cabbage have a moderate to low calcium con-

Key points

- Restricted protein levels are only recommended in patients with later stages of renal failure.
- Restricted salt levels are of importance and if the animal will not consume commercial diet, consider the use of phosphate binders.
- Transitional changes can be difficult, and support from the veterinary practice may be required.

CASE STUDY 18.1

A 16-year-old lurcher was presented to the practice for a senior health clinic. During the process of the clinic it was identified that the dog had a raised urea (15.8 mmol/l) and creatinine (204 µmol/l). The dog was therefore placed on to a renal diet. The dog suffered from severe diarrhoea when placed on this diet, despite a prolonged transitional period. It was discovered that the fat content of the renal diet was too high for this dog to digest correctly. The addition of a high-fibre diet, mixed 50 : 50, proved to be the balancing ratio. This can be a common problem with renal cases, due to the decrease in protein levels and subsequent increase in fat content.

CASE STUDY 18.2

A 3-year-old Burmese cat with a history of chronic renal failure presented with clinical symptoms of hypokalaemia. Initial blood potassium levels showed to be 2.8 mmol/l (normal range 3.5–5.8 mmol/l). The cat was placed on potassium supplements, with regular blood electrolyte analysis every 3 months. The cat was difficult to medicate on occasions, and the use of pilchards in tomato ketchup was recommended, due to the high potassium levels in the ketchup. Regular sampling was required, as the blood results show (Table 18.2) that the blood potassium levels could not be adequately stabilized. The cat was later euthanized on humane grounds at the owner's request.

tent, and make them suitable for rabbits suffering from CRF. Foodstuffs such as alfalfa, kale and broccoli have high calcium contents.

LOWER URINARY TRACT SYSTEM

CANINE UROLITHIASIS

Urolithiasis is considered to be a common disorder of the urinary tract in dogs. Clinical signs of urolithiasis may be the first indication of an underlying systemic disorder, or defect in the structure or function of the urinary tract.[8] As with feline lower urinary tract disease (see below), urolithiasis should not be viewed as a single disease process, but rather as a sequel of underlying abnormalities. Examination of the urolith composition will aid in determining the

Table 18.2 Serum potassium levels and corresponding supplements required

Sampling interval	Potassium levels (mmol/l)	Supplement levels
Initial diagnosing sample	2.8	4 scoops daily (2 b.i.d.)
1 month later	4.47	4 scoops daily (2 b.i.d.)
1 month later	3.04	6 scoops daily (3 b.i.d.)
1 month later	3.41	6 scoops daily (3 b.i.d.)
1 month later	2.86	8 scoops daily (4 b.i.d.)

aetiology. A full dietary history is required, along with analysis of serum and urine for the concentration of calculogenic minerals, crystallization promoters and crystallization inhibitors. Because of the several types of urolith that occur in dogs, each will be discussed individually, as most require different treatments and managements (Table 18.3). Urinary diets for dogs (and cats) can be divided into those that promote dissolution through changing the pH of the urine and those that act by diluting the concentration of the urine. In all cases, dietary management should only commence once obstruction (if present) has been resolved.

Nutritional aims are as follows:

- Decrease the amount of calculogenic materials within the urine.
- Increase water intake.
- Promote an optimal pH; this is dependent on the urolith present.
- Help the animal obtain its ideal weight and BCS.

Clinical nutrition
Water
Water intake is a vital factor in dogs with, or those that have a predisposition to, canine urolithiasis. The solute load of the diet influences total water intake by a large factor, the same as with cats. The use of a moist diet is preferred, and additional water can also be mixed in if required. Encouragement to increase the consumption of water can also be achieved by increasing access, by placing more bowls of water around the dog's environment. Bottled, pre-boiled water or water that has been left to stand will have little or no chlorine that can be detected by the dog. Some dogs will also play with/eat ice cubes, especially useful in the warm weather, or drink water that is flavoured. Further details are provided in Appendix 4.

Increases in water consumption will increase the total volume of urine produced. Crystals precipitate out into the urine when supersaturation occurs. Urine becomes saturated when its dissolved salt concentration cannot be exceeded. Any additional salt or a decrease in the relative fluid volume will result in precipitation of the salts; urine at this stage is said to be supersaturated. Supersaturation of the urine is the initial stage of crystal urolith formation (Fig. 18.1). Although urine supersaturation is fundamental for urolithogenesis, the whole process is complex and multifactorial. Owners are recommended that the animal's urine should remain dilute and have no strong smell. Bitches' urine does bleach/kill the grass where urination commonly occurs, but this does not reflect that crystals or uroliths are present. The use of filtered water in hard-water areas can aid in reducing the intake of minerals.

Urinalysis should be preformed on a regular basis, at least every 6 months, once placed on a long-term urinary tract diet. Sediment analysis along with pH and specific gravity are all good indicators of overall health. Fresh urine samples should be used when performing urinalysis. Samples obtained via cystocentesis should be used when obtaining samples for bacterial culture and sensitivity, especially important in dogs with suspected struvite or calcium phosphate uroliths. Urination should be

Table 18.3 Urolith formations and treatments, with urinary pH preferences[9]

Type of urolith	Urinary pH during formation	Target urinary pH	Treatment
Struvite	Alkaline	5.9–6.3	Calculolytic diet or surgical removal
Calcium oxalate	Variable but usually acidic	7.1–7.7	Surgical removal
Ammonium urate	Acidic	7.1–7.7	Calculolytic diet and allopurinol
Cystine	Acidic	7.1–7.7	Calculolytic diet or surgical removal
Silicate	Usually acidic	7.1–7.7	Surgical removal

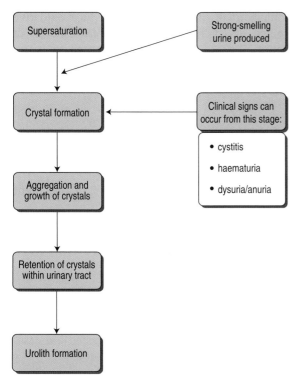

Figure 18.1 Systematic diagram of urolith and crystal formation within the urine.

encouraged as often as possible. Exercise in dogs can increase the frequency of urination.

Urate uroliths

Dalmatians have a high risk factor for recurrent urate uroliths, high enough that prophylactic therapy should be actively considered for this breed. Some texts state that Dalmatians are more susceptible as they lack the enzyme uricase, which converts uric acid to allantoin. Their urine therefore contains higher levels of urates than that of other breeds.[9] In other texts[10,11] uric acid metabolism is not considered to be affected by the absence of hepatic uricase, with uricase enzyme levels being comparable to that in other breeds. The cause has been attributed to the impaired transport of uric acid into the hepatocytes, which may reduce the rate of hepatic oxidation. Another factor can be attributed to the proximal renal tubules of Dalmatians reabsorbing less and secreting more urate than in the kidneys of other breeds of dogs.[10]

Nutrition aims of dietary management of urate urolithiasis include:

- restricting protein level
- increasing the source of non-protein calories
- promoting an alkaline urine pH.

Clinical nutrition
Proteins
A diet designed to aid in urate urolithiasis should have restricted levels of proteins (1.6–2.2 g protein/ 100 kcal metabolizable energy (ME)),[11] especially those proteins that contain larger amounts of nucleic acids, as they contain purines, e.g. protein from muscle or organ tissues. Milk proteins (casein) and eggs provide a suitable source, as they contain a lower amount of purines, but also have a high biological value, which is required when restriction of protein levels is required in the diet.

Allopurinol needs to be added to the diet when dissolution of urate uroliths is required, though checking the dietary manufacturer's guidelines is recommended. Allopurinol is a xanthine oxidase inhibitor, which reduces the rate of urate excretion into the urine. A dose rate of 15 mg/kg orally b.i.d. should be utilized, though dose rate is dependent on the individual.

Carbohydrates and fats
Because of the restriction in protein levels, it is important that there is a sufficient supply of non-protein calories. A higher than normal fat content can arise from this, and care should be given to control of the animal's weight. The level of fats also aids in obtaining the preferred urine pH.

Vitamins and minerals
As with any disease or disorder in which clinical symptoms include polyuria, the water-soluble vitamins should be supplemented. However, in urolithiasis, vitamin C should not be supplemented, as it is a precursor of oxalate, and can predispose to its formation.

The alkalizing agents used in these diets are commonly potassium citrate and calcium carbonate. If the target urinary pH is not reached, then additional potassium citrate can be added to the diet at a starting dose rate of 50–100 mg/kg BW orally b.i.d., until the pH of the urine reaches the desired level.[11]

Struvite uroliths

Struvite uroliths in dogs, as in cats, are the most commonly occurring uroliths, though their incidence rate is decreasing. Infection-induced struvite uroliths are common in dogs. Antimicrobial therapy should be initiated alongside nutritional management, if urinalysis proves to be positive upon culturing. The bacteria present tend to be urease-producing staphylococci.

Nutritional aims of dietary management of struvite uroliths include:

- dissolution of uroliths within the bladder
- preventing the formation of reoccurring uroliths or crystals
- promoting an acidic urine pH.

Clinical nutrition
Proteins
Restricted levels of protein are required (1.47 g protein/100 kcal ME), but a high biological value is needed. When protein levels are this restricted, it is not advisable to be fed this diet long term. The urine acidifying substance in diets designed for struvite dissolution is DL-methionine, used at a dose rate of 0.5 g/kg of diet.

Carbohydrates
The majority of calories obtained from the diet need to be obtained from a non-protein source. Thus, the carbohydrate and fat levels are increased in these diets.

Fats
Struvite diets can have very high fat levels (~26% DM), so much so that in some brands only tinned formulas are available. Feeding diets with this high a fat content to dogs with hyperlipidaemia, pancreatitis or even at-risk groups is contraindicated.

Vitamins and minerals
Decreased amounts of phosphorus (24 mg phosphorus/100 kcal ME) and magnesium (3.3 mg magnesium/100 kcal ME) are present in these diets, as these are the constituents of the urolith. Sodium levels are often increased, in order to increase water intake (23.3 mg sodium/100 kcal ME). The antioxidants, vitamin E and beta-carotene, are often supplemented, as this helps to reduce oxidative damage, and helps combat urolithiasis. Levels of vitamin C should not be supplemented, as it is a precursor of oxalate, which can form when feeding diets designed for struvite dissolution.

Calcium oxalate uroliths

Calcium oxalate uroliths are the second most commonly occurring uroliths in the dog.

Nutritional aims of dietary management include:

- promoting an alkaline urinary pH
- reducing the amounts of calcium, sodium and oxalates within the diet.

Clinical nutrition
Protein
A low-protein diet is required, with levels of 1.6–2.2 g/100 kcal ME having been suggested[11] in cases where calcium oxalate uroliths are present.

Fats and carbohydrates
Non-protein calories are required in the diet, in order to prevent protein catabolism. Thus, levels of fats and carbohydrates are higher than normal. Weight management can be a problem in dogs that are predisposed to weight gain.

Vitamins and minerals
Neither vitamin D nor C should be supplemented in the diet. Vitamin D increases the absorption of calcium from the diet, whereas vitamin C acts as a precursor to oxalates. The levels of calcium in the diet should be restricted, but not reduced, as with levels of sodium. Sodium increases calcium excretion into the urine, and a dietary level of 0.1–0.2% sodium DMB or 45–55 mg sodium/100 kcal ME is recommended.[11]

Cystine urolithiasis

Cystine uroliths are uncommon in both cats and dogs, but arise due to a metabolic defect where the reabsorption of filtered cystine in the proximal tube is impaired.[12] Once in the urine, cystine is very insoluble, especially in acidic urine.

Nutritional aims in the management of cystine uroliths include:

- promoting an alkaline urine pH
- reducing the amount of cystine produced by the body.

Clinical nutrition
Protein
A low-protein diet is required (9–11% protein DMB), as this will aid in the reduction of the total daily excretion of cystine.

Carbohydrates and fats
Because of the low levels of protein in the diet, calories have to be obtained from these nutrients.

Vitamins and minerals
Low sodium levels are also required, as sodium excretion can enhance cystine excretion. Low sodium in combination with low protein levels tends to increase the urine volume, which further decreases the urinary concentration of cystine.[11] In order to create an alkaline urine pH, supplementation with oral potassium citrate (50–100 mg/kg BW b.i.d.) is required.

Silicate uroliths

These uroliths are more commonly seen in male dogs (96%) than in females (4%).[8] This is most likely due to females being able to pass smaller uroliths before they can induce clinical signs. Foods that contain large amounts of plant-derived materials are thought to be a predisposing factor for silicate uroliths. Another factor is the consumption of soil.

Dietary management of dogs suffering from silicate uroliths aims at prevention. A diet that does not contain large amounts of plant-derived material, and increases the volume of urine produced, will help control the main factors. Debate has arisen over urinary pH levels; alkalization of the urine in order to increase the solubility of silica is unknown.[13]

Feeding a dog with urolithiasis

Nearly all diets aimed at dissolution or prevention of uroliths are high in fat, mainly because of the requirement for non-protein calories. Care should be given when transferring a dog over to these diets. Caution should also be used with dogs that are likely to gain weight, or those that are predisposed to hyperlipidaemia or pancreatitis. Diarrhoea can occur when high fat levels are fed, and combination with a high-fibre diet that is aimed at urolith prevention may be required.

Calculolytic diets are only successful when fed alone. Addition of treats and home-cooked foods can undo the desired effect of the diet. It is equally important that the urolith analysis is correct. Stones that are of mixed composition are difficult to dissolve, and surgical removal may be the treatment of choice. In dogs suffering from struvite urolithiasis, if you have the suspicion that additional snacks or treats are being fed, a blood sample analysis can be useful. In dogs being fed certain veterinary struvite dissolution diets, a low plasma urea concentration of less than 4 mmol/l (BUN 10 mg/dl) is found. A value above this levels suggests additional feeding.

Monitoring of dogs suffering from urolithiasis is vital. Urinalysis should be performed at least every 6 months once dissolution has occurred. Preventative measures involve feeding a diet that promotes the correct urine pH, provides calories from a non-protein source and is relatively low in the salts that are the building blocks for the uroliths from which the animal suffers.

Key points

- Regular urinalysis while on the diet, including pH monitoring and microscopy, is vital.
- Regular weight checks.
- Prevention in at-risk breeds outweighs cure.
- Increase water intake as much as possible in all groups.

FELINE LOWER URINARY TRACT DISEASE (FLUTD)

Feline lower urinary tract disease (FLUTD) is becoming more prevalent in the feline population, possibly due to an increase in the number of animals with

CASE STUDY 18.3

An 11-year-old bichon frise had undergone a cystotomy due to the presence of oxalate uroliths. In this case six points of action were recommended and undertaken:

- Place on a prescription diet for uroliths, and avoid foods that contain milk, fish, cheese, etc.
- Increase water consumption.
- Take regular urine samples, checking urine pH (should be 7.1–7.7).
- Measure blood calcium levels.
- Culture urine for any bacterial infection.
- Avoid obesity.

The dog was overweight, 11.5 kg (ideal 10 kg), and advice was given regarding exercise regimens and the dog was placed on a prescription veterinary diet. As the diet is low in protein, and calories are obtained from the higher fat contents, digestion can be a problem in some dogs. In this case the dog's faeces were very soft, and causing the owner concern, as the fur was becoming matted around the anus. It was recommended that the owner mix in a high-fibre diet that can also be recommended for dogs suffering from uroliths. Adjustments in the proportions of diets were required until the diarrhoea was resolved. Urinalysis showed that even though the dog was on the correct diet, the urine pH was still at 5–6. Potassium citrate was required in order to help alkalinize the urine, at a dose rate of 50–150 mg/kg. A mid range of 1000 mg/day was administered, with urinalysis again occurring on a regular basis until optimal urine pH was achieved.

Table 18.4   Risk factors associated with increases in FLUTD cases

Age	Most commonly seen in cats between 1–10 years
Gender	Males and females have a similar risk of non-obstructive FLUTD. Prevalence of urethral obstruction is more common in males
Neuter status	Neutering in both males and females is associated with an increase in risk
Food	An increase in dry food consumption can increase risk factor
Weight	Excessive weight (obesity) will increase the risk of FLUTD
Water consumption	A decrease in water consumption can greatly increase the risk
Activity levels	Animals that have a more sedentary lifestyle are more likely to develop FLUTD
Weather conditions	Veterinary practices are more likely to see an increase in FLUTD cases when the weather is poor, possibly because cats are unwilling to urinate outdoors in wet weather

increased risk factors (Table 18.4). FLUTD accounts for approximately 7% of feline cases presented to veterinary practices. It may result from a number of different aetiologies including infection, neoplasia, urolithiasis, neurological disorders, anatomical abnormalities and inflammatory conditions.

Urine is a complex solution of both organic and inorganic ions. Crystals can grow and form when an imbalance occurs in this solution. There are several factors that can cause these imbalances. Diet, decreased water consumption, urine pH alterations or relative lack of inhibitors of crystallization can cause the solubility of a particular crystal to be exceeded. This results in crystal aggregation and growth. Clinical signs of FLUTD include haematuria, proteinuria, dysuria, pollakiuria (extraordinary urinary frequency), and/or urethral obstruction.[14]

Dietary manipulation can aid in reducing the risk factors for uroliths. Nutritional aims of diets aimed at FLUTD vary because of the multifactorial nature of the disease. Aims include:

- Increasing the solubility of the products. This is achieved by obtaining a urinary pH, which will dissolve any crystals that have formed in the urine, and aid in prevention of any further crystal formation.
- Eliminating or reducing the risk of supersaturation.
- Increasing the presence of inhibitors of crystallization.
- Aiding the animal to obtain an ideal body condition score if required.

Struvite crystals

Struvite crystals ($MgNH_4PO_4.6H_2O$) (Fig. 18.2) are commonly seen in cats suffering from FLUTD. Dietary recommendations for these cats include avoiding excessive dietary protein, and avoiding excessive levels of the minerals that occur within the crystals (magnesium and phosphorus). Urinary pH needs to be acidic, as the crystals form in an alkaline environment. A range of 5.9–6.1 is ideal for dissolution, whereas 6.2–6.4 is recommended for prevention. The average urinary pH of a domestic cat consuming a natural diet (small rodents) is 6.3. Acidifiers are used to prevent struvite uroliths. Cats receiving long-term dietary acidifiers can suffer from a transient negative potassium balance with phosphoric acid and ammonium chloride acidifiers. Long-term potassium depletion will stimulate ammonia synthesis at the same time as chronic metabolic acidosis. Acidifying therapeutic veterinary diets need to have potassium levels in excess of the National Research Council (NRC) minimum allowance of 0.6% (DMB).[15] The use of urinary acidifiers alongside an acidifying food is not recommended, as it can lead to metabolic acidosis. The alterations in pH may increase the solubility of some of the solutes within the urine, and in some cases decrease the solubility of others. This complex and competing interplay between nutritional requirements of the management of oxalate and struvite urolithiasis requires a careful selection in the long-term dietary control of FLUTD.

Oxalate crystals

The nutritional management of cats suffering from oxalate crystals differs in that the aim is to achieve a less acidic urinary pH of 6.6–6.8. Citrate is commonly supplemented in diets specifically for cats suffering from oxalate crystals (Fig. 18.3) or uroliths. The citrate increases the urinary pH, and forms soluble complexes with the calcium, thereby inhibiting calcium oxalate formation.

Clinical nutrition

Water

Water intake is a vital factor in cats with FLUTD or a predisposition to FLUTD. The solute load of the diet influences total water intake by a large factor. Use of a moist diet is preferred, and additional water can also be mixed in if required. Encouragement to increase the consumption of water can also be achieved by increasing access, by placing more bowls of water around the cat's environment. The choice of type and size of water bowls needs to be considered. Cats can be deterred by the use of fresh tap water because of the chlorine content. Bottled, pre-boiled water or water that has been left to stand will have little or no chlorine that can be detected by the cat. Further details are provided in Appendix 4.

Increased intake of water is necessary to avoid supersaturation of the urine and the precipitation of crystals (see p. 160). The urine of the cat, like that of the dog, should be dilute and have no strong smell. Analysis of fresh urine samples should be carried out at least every 6 months, and those for bacterial culture and sensitivity should be obtained by cystocentesis. Voided samples and those not examined immediately can have false positives for bacteria and crystalluria.

Protein

Excessive levels of protein need to be avoided in cases where struvite crystals and alkaline urine are present. High protein levels can influence pH; a prime example of this is the difference in urine pH

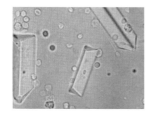

Figure 18.2 Struvite crystals.

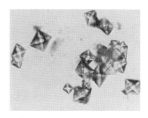

Figure 18.3 Oxalate crystals.

between cats and dogs. Cats have higher protein consumption than dogs, and therefore an increased urinary pH. Increasing the protein level in the diet also increases urinary calcium excretion, uric acid and oxalate excretion. Excess dietary protein should be avoided by feeding a food that contains 30–45% DM protein.[15]

Fats

Diets that promote urinary tract health do tend to have a higher fat content. This is due to the increased energy density which overall reduces mineral intake. When metabolized, fat produces the highest metabolic water contribution, which also benefits the animal. Owing to the increased fat content, some veterinary therapeutic diets are not available in a dry form. Obesity is a major risk factor of FLUTD, and a diet with a higher fat content may not be the indicated diet in this circumstance.

Carbohydrates

Cats that suffer from FLUTD and are overweight need to be placed on an obesity diet, many of which have higher fibre content. The quantity of calcium being absorbed from the digestive system can be reduced by certain sources of dietary fibre. This can be beneficial with cats suffering from recurrent calcium oxalate urolithiasis.

Vitamins and minerals

Struvite precipitates when the urine becomes supersaturated with magnesium, anionic phosphate and ammonium. Therapeutic diets avoid excess dietary magnesium, but low urinary magnesium concentrations have the potential to increase the risk of formation of calcium-containing uroliths, highlighting the importance of regular urinalysis when on a therapeutic urinary diet. The intake of magnesium and calcium also influences urinary phosphate concentrations (Tables 18.5 and 18.6).

The addition of sodium to the diet is occasionally used to aid in increased water intake. Increasing the salt content of the diet can aid in diuresis and lowers the urine specific gravity. Sodium, however, does increase calcium excretion into the urine, thus increasing the risk of calcium-based uroliths (e.g. oxalate). Increased sodium levels are also discouraged in older animals, because of a possibility of decreased renal function. Recent links have been

made to the occurrence of CRF in cats that have previously suffered from FLUTD. A sodium level of 1.2% (DMB) has proven to present a health risk to cats when being fed at this level long term.[16] Added antioxidants can help combat urolithiasis, by reducing oxidative cell damage.

Supplements

The use of nutraceuticals in cases of FLUTD is commonplace. Glycoaminoglycans (GAGs) and chondroitin are widely used in order to provide a protective lining to the bladder. In the healthy animal there is a GAG layer that lines the urothelium in the bladder, and contributes towards the protection of the bladder wall from substances (e.g. crystals) present within the urine. Cats suffering from FLUTD can have a decreased excretion of urinary GAGs, and deficiencies in the GAG layer can contribute to urothelial damage, and ulceration and inflammation of the bladder wall.[16] The edges of the crystals can cause trauma to the lining of the bladder, resulting in haematuria. These types of nutraceuticals do not prevent reoccurrence of the crystals, but help to prevent reoccurrence of some of the clinical signs. Evaluation of treatment should be made over a sufficient period of time (e.g. 3–6 months).

Feeding a cat with FLUTD

The choice of diet is dependent on two factors, the body condition of the animal and results of the urinalysis. Correct identification of the type of crystals present (if any) and the pH of the urine is necessary. Use of a diet that promotes urinary health tends to be aimed at preventing struvite formation. Use of these diets in cats with a predisposition to calcium oxalate uroliths may increase the risk of urolith formation. It should be noted that the prevalence of oxalate uroliths has been increasing with a subsequent decrease in struvite uroliths. A full dietary history of the cat is required, including any treats, or supplements (especially if containing calcium), and whether or not the owner gives the cat milk. Both treats and processed human food (processed meats) are high in mineral levels, such as phosphorus, and should be avoided.

Table 18.5 Recommended levels of minerals in commercial cat foods used for dissolution and prevention of struvite uroliths

Nutrient	% Dry matter		Caloric basis (per 100 kcal)	
	Preventative	Dissolution	Preventative	Dissolution
Phosphorus	0.5–0.9	0.5–0.8	0.11–0.24 g	0.11–0.17 g
Sodium	0.2–0.6	0.7–0.9	0.06–0.11 g	0.15–0.18 g
Magnesium	0.04–0.1	0.04–0.06	9–24 g	9–12 g

Use of a moist diet is preferable, as is ad libitum feeding. This might not be possible if the cat is overweight with this feeding scenario. When any animal consumes food, gastric acid is secreted and creates a temporary net acid loss from the body, and alkalization of the urine. This is referred to as the postprandial alkaline tide. The alkaline tide is caused by secretion of bicarbonate into the blood by parietal cells of the stomach. A transient bicarbonization is produced and increases urinary pH. Acidifiers in the diet will offset this increase in pH. If the diet is offered free choice (ad libitum), the cat will eat little and often. These feeding habits result in a smaller but more prolonged alkaline tide. This can reduce the likelihood of struvite precipitate formation.

Recommendations should be given to clients about preventative measures in all cats. There are clear risk factors associated with FLUTD; some such as age, breed and gender cannot be helped, others such as lifestyle and obesity can. Neutering has a significant impact on the risk of bladder stones, the risk of oxalate increasing sevenfold, struvite 3.5-fold.[17] Educating the owner to ensure an adequate water intake, and limiting weight gain after neutering is vital.

Table 18.6 Recommended levels of minerals in commercial cat foods used for dissolution of calcium-containing uroliths

Nutrient	% Dry matter	Caloric basis (per 100 kcal)
Calcium	0.5–0.8	0.11–0.2 g
Phosphorus	0.5–0.7	0.1–0.16 g
Sodium	0.1–0.4	0.03–0.1 g
Magnesium	0.04–0.1	18–20 mg

Key points

- Increase water intake, and thus urinary dilution.
- Perform regular urinalysis, even once dissolution has been achieved. It should also be recommended that full blood haematology and biochemistry be performed on a regular basis, because of the link between FLUTD and renal failure in older cats.
- Educate clients to take preventative measures against the formation of urinary calculi throughout a cat's life, starting from a young age.
- Maintain a urinary pH of 6–6.5 in healthy cats, where dissolution is not required.

CASE STUDY 18.4

A 6-year-old male neutered cat was presented with haematuria and dysuria. The cat was grossly overweight, 9.8 kg (ideal weight 5 kg), and had a BCS of 5/5. Microscopy of the urine showed large amounts of struvite crystals, and erythrocytes. Blood samples were taken to confirm renal function prior to placing the cat onto NSAIDs. A course of antibiotics was also implemented. The cat was placed on a weight-reduction diet, which also aids in the dissolution of the struvite crystals. Water consumption also had to be dramatically increased in this cat, and thus a moist diet was used along with suggestions in Appendix 4. The cat's activity levels also needed to be increased, and the owner was advised to place the cat's food in different places so that it had to go find the food, and toys were also introduced.

The cat was monitored regularly for weight loss, and urinalysis routinely carried out every 6 months.

RABBIT UROLITHIASIS

Rabbits excrete higher levels of calcium in their urine than other mammals, and this contributes towards the cloudiness of the urine. Haematuria can also be incorrectly diagnosed in rabbits. Many rabbit caretakers and uninformed veterinary personnel mistake the orange-to-red coloured by-products in the urine (porphyrinuria) for blood. These by-products result from chlorophyll and other vegetable components. Calcium carbonate crystals are considered normal in the urine, but can easily become a problem when stones are formed. Clinical symptoms of bladder disease and/or bladder stones will vary in each individual, but can include:

- urine scalding
- wetness around the genital area
- semi-solid urine – can be described as toothpaste-like
- dysuria, demonstrated by hopping in and out of the litter tray/pan, straining and loss of litter training.

Diagnosis can be easily made with radiography and urinalysis, though it should be remembered that rabbits will have some radio-opaque material present in the urine due to its high calcium content. The only treatment for calcium-containing uroliths is surgery; they cannot be dissolved.

Clinical nutrition

Clinical nutrition for these animals is based on the reduction of calcium in the diet, and perioperative nutrition. This again is dependent on the nutritional status of the individual animal. Lowering blood calcium levels is a simpler process than in other mammals. A medium-sized rabbit has a daily minimum requirement of 510 mg of calcium.[18] Alfalfa hay is extremely high in calcium and should not be fed to these animals. The use of grass hays, such as timothy or oat hay is advocated. Root vegetables are low in calcium, but the majority of vegetables fed to rabbits tend to have high calcium contents. These greens should be cut down on, but not removed, as they are still a very important component of the diet. Broccoli flowers and stem, dark leaf lettuce, watercress, Brussels sprouts, celery leaves, and cabbage are good choices when trying to reduce calcium. Pelleted diets should also be removed or restricted; pellets designed for young rabbits, or those containing alfalfa, should be avoided.

References

1. Lane IF. Nutritional management of urinary tract conditions. In: Ettinger SJ, Feldman EC, eds. Textbook of veterinary internal medicine. Volume 1. 6th edn. St Louis, Missouri: Elsevier Saunders; 2005:584–586.
2. Allen TA, Polzin DJ, Adams LG. Renal disease. In: Hand MS, Thatcher CD, Remillard RL, et al., eds. Small animal clinical nutrition. 4th edn. Missouri: Mark Morris Institute; 2000:563–604.
3. Robertson JL, Goldschmidt M, Kronfeld DS, et al. Long-term renal responses to high dietary protein in dogs with 75% nephrectomy. Kidney Int 1986; 29:511–519.
4. Elliott DA. Nutritional management of chronic renal disease. Waltham Focus 2005; 15(1):14–19.
5. Elliott J, Rawlings JM, Markwell PJ, et al. Survival of cats with naturally occurring chronic renal failure: effect of dietary management. J Small Anim Pract 2000; 41:235–242.
6. Plantinga EA, Everts H, Kastelein AMC, et al. Retrospective study of the survival of cats with acquired chronic renal insufficiency offered different commercial diets. Vet Rec 2005; 157:185–187.
7. Harcourt-Brown F. Anorexia in rabbits 2: Diagnosis and treatment. In Practice 2002; (Sept):450–467.
8. Osborne CA, Bartges JW, Lulich JP, et al. Canine urolithiasis. In: Hand MS, Thatcher CD, Remillard RL, et al., eds. Small animal clinical nutrition. 4th edn. Missouri: Mark Morris Institute; 2000:605–688.
9. Agar S. Small animal nutrition. Edinburgh: Butterworth-Heinemann; 2003.
10. Buffington CAT, Holloway C, Abood SK. Manual of veterinary dietetics. Missouri: Elsevier Saunders; 2004.

11. Senior DF. Urolithiasis – a nutritional perspective. In: Kelly N, Wills J, eds. BSAVA manual of companion animal nutrition and feeding. Gloucester: BSAVA Publications; 1996:188–197.

12. Bovee KC. Genetic and metabolic diseases of the kidney. In: Bovee KC, ed. Canine nephrology. Pennsylvania: Harwell Publications; 1984: 339–354.

13. Osborne CA, Clinton CW, Kim KM. Etiopathogenesis, clinical manifestations and management of silica urolithiasis. Vet Clin Small Anim 1986; 161:85–207.

14. Gunn-Moore DA. Update on feline lower urinary tract disease. Watford: Ceva Animal Health Ltd; 2000.

15. Kirk CA. Dietary salt and FLUTD: risk or benefit? Proceedings of the 20th Annual ACUIM Forum; 2000:553–555.

16. Sparkes A. Urolithiasis in cats: optimum management to prevent recurrence. Veterinary Review 2006; 115:20–28.

17. Lekcharoensuk C, Lulich JP, Osborne CA. Association between patients related factors and risk of calcium oxalate and magnesium ammonium phosphate urolithiasis in cats. J Am Vet Med Assoc 2000; 217(4):520–525.

18. Harkness JE. Summary of calcium in rabbits. Rabbit Health News 1994; 11:7.

Suggested reading (clinical nutrition)

Agar S. Small animal nutrition. Edinburgh: Butterworth-Heinemann; 2003.

Buffington T, Holloway C, Abood S. Manual of veterinary dietetics. St Louis, Missouri: Elsevier Saunders; 2004.

Burger I. The Waltham book of companion animal nutrition. Oxford: Pergamon Press; 1993.

Frape D. Equine nutrition and feeding. 2nd edn. Oxford: Blackwell Science; 1998.

Hand MS, Thatcher CD, Remillard RL, et al., eds. Small animal clinical nutrition. 4th edn. Missouri: Mark Morris Institute; 2000.

Higgins AJ, Wright IM, eds. The equine manual. London: Saunders; 1995.

section 5

Avian and Reptile Nutrition

19

Avian nutrition

Water

Water, as in all animals, is a vital part of nutrition and should be available at all times. Anyone who has cared for a bird will know that the provision of fresh clean water is difficult, because contamination of the drinking water with food and faeces is common. Subclinical bacterial infections are associated with contaminated water bowls. Some birds can easily adapt to the use of water bottles, and this behaviour should be encouraged.

The water source should also be considered. Tap water can have a higher mineral content, depending on geographical location. Iron content can differ greatly, and can be detrimental to those birds that suffer from haemochromatosis (iron storage disease).

Diet

The diet of birds is specific for each breed, and should be adequately researched for each patient. The use of complete pelleted diets is becoming more popular and should be recommended to owners, as it reduces selective feeding. Fresh fruit and vegetables should be available to birds, but correctly washed and prepared. Seed diets can be deficient in many nutrients (Table 19.1), and are commonly fortified with vitamin and mineral supplements. Problems can arise when the bird hulls the shell from the seed, and the nutrients are lost. Table 19.2 notes clinical symptoms of vitamin and mineral deficiencies in birds.

It has been shown that many species of birds, especially budgerigars and cockatiels, are prone to renal disease if they are fed a 100% pelleted diet, or seed diet long term.[1] It is therefore recommended

Table 19.1 **Essential dietary nutrients deficient in seeds[2]**

Dietary nutrient class	Specific nutrient deficiency
Vitamins	Vitamin A, choline, niacin, pantothenic acid, riboflavin (B$_2$), cyanocobalamine (B$_{12}$), biotin, folic acid, D, E and K
Minerals	Calcium, phosphorus, sodium
Trace minerals	Selenium, iron, copper, zinc, manganese, iodine, chromium, vanadium, bismuth, tin and boron
Pigments	Chlorophyll and canthexanine
Essential amino acids	Lysine and methionine
Fibre	Mucopolysaccharides, both soluble and insoluble fibre
Vitamin precursors	Beta carotene (converted to vitamin A in the liver)
Fatty acids	Omega fatty acids

Table 19.2 **Vitamin and mineral deficiencies in birds**

Vitamin or mineral	Clinical symptoms of deficiency
A	Squamous metaplasia, loss of choanal papillae, oral abscesses and pododermatitis
D	Weakness, muscle tremors and fitting
E	Muscle dystrophies of the skeletal system and cardiac muscle, as well as encephalomalacia and exudative diathesis
K	Causes prolongation of clotting times
Thiamin (B$_1$)	Inappetence, opisthotonus, seizures and death
Riboflavin (B$_2$)	Weakness, diarrhoea, curled toe paralysis, feathering abnormalities
Niacin	Stomatitis, poor feathering, diarrhoea, some leg deformities
Pyridoxine (B$_6$)	Inappetence, perosis, jerky movements, poor growth
Pantothenic acid	Poor feathering, dermatitis, perosis and ataxia
Biotin	Poor feathering, dermatitis, perosis and ataxia
Folic acid	Leg deformities, beak deformities, poor growth and embryonic death
Choline	Poor growth, feather abnormalities
Vitamin C	Not yet documented

that a small percentage of pellets and a small percentage of seeds (Box 19.1), especially millet and sprouted seeds, are given alongside a wide range of fresh foods. Examples of good fresh foods to use include bread, cooked pasta, brown rice, legumes, fruit and vegetables. The use of sprouting seeds should be advocated. The process of sprouting utilizes some of the seeds' fat stores, whilst helping to accustom the bird to vegetables. In order for a bird to feed, it must feel comfortable in its environment (Fig. 19.1). This is especially important during diet conversions, and during periods of stress.

required, but the root cause of the hypervitaminosis should be addressed. Initial treatment is vitamin A 10–15 IU/g, and then a maintenance dose of 0.25 IU/g. Treatment of any secondary infections needs to be investigated. Seed mixes can be vitamin fortified, but the vitamins are usually on the shell. When the seed is hulled, the fortification is lost.

Hypocalcaemia

Hypocalcaemia is a recognized syndrome in grey parrots, and although the aetiology is unconfirmed seed-based diets have been proposed as the cause. This is due to the low calcium and vitamin D_3 concentrations within these diets. Hyperparathyroidism may also have a role to play.[3] The role of UV light (285–315 nm wavelength) plays an integral part in the synthesis of vitamin D_3 and thus the absorption of calcium. Birds that are housed indoors can receive inadequate levels of UV light, even if housed by a window. Glass filters out the necessary UV light for cutaneous synthesis.

Low ionized calcium results in a decrease in electrical resistance and an increase in membrane permeability (to sodium and potassium) of nerve tissue. This results in hyperexcitability of muscle and neural tissue. High-protein diets and acidification of the intestines aids in calcium absorption; seed diets are high in fat and directly influence the intestinal concentration of free fatty acids. The high free fatty acids and a possibility of impaired fat digestion will result in the formation of insoluble calcium soaps. A full dietary history is required, as some foodstuffs contain compounds such as oxalates (found in spinach and rhubarb), phylate (in cereal grains) and phosphates that form complexes with the calcium and decrease absorption. The ratio of calcium to available phosphorus is approximately 2:1; ranges of 0.5:1 to 2.5:1 can be tolerated but as this ratio moves away from the ideal, the more critical vitamin D levels become.[3] Over-supplementation of calcium can be detrimental; levels of over 1.0% calcium in the diet can lead to a decrease in the utilization of proteins, fats, vitamins, phosphorus, magnesium, iron, iodine, zinc and manganese. When marginal intakes of one or more of these nutrients occur the increase in calcium can induce a deficiency.

When monitoring calcium levels, both ionized and free calcium should be requested in blood samples.

Box 19.1 Sunflower vs safflower seeds

Many texts, internet sites and pet stores recommend the use of safflower seeds rather than sunflower, within a bird's diet. Both seeds are high in fat, whilst having limited other nutrients. Contrary to previous thought, sunflower seeds do not possess any addictive ingredients. Safflower seeds are slightly bitter tasting in comparison to sunflower seeds, and this is why birds prefer sunflower seeds.[1]

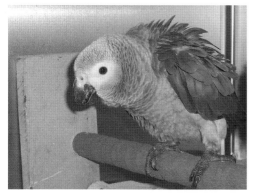

Figure 19.1 Hospitalized birds require a stimulating environment in which to feed and feel comfortable.

Commonly observed malnutrition

Hypovitaminosis A

Hypovitaminosis A is the most common problem seen in birds that primarily consume a seed diet, mainly in parrots and other large psittacines. Clinical symptoms include the choanal papillae being blunt or absent, and lesions of *Candida* spp. Initially, nasal discharge and coughing are present, followed by lethargy. Diagnosis can be made on these clinical symptoms and by obtaining a detailed history, including diet and husbandry. Resolution of clinical symptoms is rapid with treatment. Parenteral administration of vitamin A is commonly utilized, but toxicity of vitamin A if over-supplemented should be noted. Oral administration of beta-carotene, vitamin A's precursor, is a safer option. The bird can convert required amounts of vitamin A from the beta-carotene and excrete the rest. Supplementing the diet with vitamin A may be

Protein and essential amino acid (EAA) deficiency

When consuming a diet with poor protein quality, higher levels of protein need to be consumed in order to obtain the required nutrients. This can lead to a total excessive consumption of proteins. Any deficiency will lead to poor growth rates, a reduction in fertility, and poor health. Excessive proteins need to be eliminated through utilization as an energy source, which may result in obesity or in gout due to the formation of urates. In many avian diets lysine is the amino acid that has the lowest levels, and is thus most frequently deficient. The lack of lysine in the diet can lead to a reduced optimal use of the other amino acids, methionine, arginine, tryptophan and threonine. Problems associated with excess protein are often also linked to calcium. High levels of both protein and calcium are often associated with stunting, whereas high levels of protein and low levels of calcium can lead to leg deformities. Gout can also be seen.

Gout

Diets excessive in protein can lead to a build-up of the primary nitrogenous metabolic product, uric acid. Uric acid is produced by the liver and excreted by the renal tubules. In birds gout can be classified as renal or articular. When uric acid reaches saturation point in the blood it will crystallize out into the membranes of the kidneys (renal gout) and/or into the joint spaces (articular gout). The pathogenesis of gout is not clear, but water deprivation and nephrosis may have a considerable effect.

Hypovitaminosis E

Vitamin E is a superb antioxidant and is commonly used in the preservation of some foods. When fats within foods become rancid vitamin E deficiency can occur. These deficiencies often occur in cockatiels, and in conjunction with selenium and sulphur-containing amino acid deficiencies.

Tube feeding birds

The passing of a tube into the crop of birds is an important technique to learn. Formulas used include critical care/recovery and neonate powders, which are now available on the market. When crop feeding it is important that the formula used is at the correct temperature. The food used should be warmed, but only to a temperature slightly lower than the bird's own body temperature. The tube should be passed over the trachea at the base of the tongue down the oesophagus and palpated in the crop at the thoracic inlet. Whilst administering the formula the back of the bird's mouth should be viewed to ensure that crop overfill does not occur. If it does, try to withdraw some of the formula with reverse suction, and withdraw the tube. The bird is better positioned to try to remove some of the formula, and to clear its own airway. Handling the bird after the administration of food or medications is not recommended, unless respiratory distress is observed.[4]

References

1. Wissman MA. The importance of avian nutrition. 2006. Online. Available: http://www.exoticpetvet.net
2. Stockdale B. Principles of avian nutrition: the theory and practice. Proceedings of the Parrot Society Meeting. 18th May 2003.
3. Stanford M. Calcium metabolism in grey parrots: the effects of husbandry. Monterey, CA: HBD International Chat AAV; 2002.
4. Tully TN. Care of birds, reptiles and small mammals. In: McCurnin DM, Bassert JM, eds. Clinical textbook for veterinary technicians. 6th edn. St Louis, Missouri: Elsevier Saunders; 2006:548–572.

20

Reptile nutrition

Reptiles present nutritional challenges. Each species has an ideal habitat, optimal ranges of temperature (preferred optimal temperature zone; POTZ) and humidity, specific preferences for food, and nutritional heritage, manifested as digestive and metabolic adaptations that directly influence its requirements for water, calories and nutrients. For example, shell deformities in tortoises are so common that some people now believe that all tortoises are meant to have lumpy shells.

Temperature

Ambient temperature is vitally important. Because these animals are exothermic, they need to be housed at a high enough temperature and correct humidity so that they can catch, eat and digest their food. The ambient temperature affects body core temperature, activity, including food procurement, and food energy needs.[1]

Energy requirements

The daily estimated energy needs for these animals are extrapolated from domestic species, based on calculations of average standard metabolic rate (SMR), usually measured on fasting animals, at rest in a dark, temperature-controlled environment.[2] Equations designed to calculate energy levels for various species are similar, even though a turtle's and tortoise's shell will comprise 15–30% of its bodyweight (Table 20.1). The energy source of choice for each species is dependent on whether the animal is a herbivore, omnivore or carnivore. Table 20.2 demonstrates the differences in diet between the different groups.

As with mammals, energy requirements increase with reproduction, growth, increased protein syn-

Table 20.1 **Daily energy requirements equations for various species**

Species	Temperature (°C)	Metabolic rate (kcal/day)*
Many, averaged	30	$32\,(BW^{0.77})$
Lizards	30	$28\,(BW^{0.83})$
Lizards	37	$48\,(BW^{0.82})$
Snakes	30	$32\,(BW^{0.76})$
Turtles	30	$32\,(BW^{0.86})$

*Standard metabolic rates were measured on fasting animals, resting in the dark in the inactive phase of a diurnal cycle.[2]

Table 20.2 **Estimated nutritional energy requirements for captive reptiles**[2]

	Dietary contents % kcal ME		
	Carnivore	*Omnivore*	*Herbivore*
Protein	25–60	15–40	15–35
Fat	30–60	5–40	< 10
Carbohydrate	< 10	20–75	55–75

ME, metabolizable energy.

thesis (as in wound healing), and with certain disorders. Fuel sources for sick reptiles often approximate usual intakes when healthy – protein and fats for carnivores and increased carbohydrates for herbivores. For patients suffering from severe trauma, infection or burns, there is an increase in metabolic rate (hypermetabolism) and a shift towards relatively more utilization of fats and proteins.[1]

Hypermetabolic patients should be fed frequent small meals of a diet that utilizes highly digestible ingredients and emphasizes protein and fat. Provision of adequate calories and protein will minimize the use of endogenous proteins as an energy source. The feeding schedules and routes of diet administration depend on the patient's metabolic state and the availability of materials, nursing care and specialist diets. Starvation can arise from many different circumstances, including stress-induced failure to eat, provision of too little food or feeding management and diseases that affect appetite and metabolism. To treat complications that arise from starvation, first restoration of fluid and electrolyte levels is vital. Digestive and metabolic upsets occur when debilitated patients only receive 40–75% of their energy requirements.[2] The patient needs to be raised gradually over 2–5 days to full nutritional goal, exactly the same as in mammals. Once this goal has been reached, nutritional support should be tapered off as voluntary food intake commences.

Water

All animals must have free access to water throughout the day. The way in which the water is provided for reptiles should be adapted for the individual species. Turtles, tortoises, snakes and many lizards will drink from bowls. Some species will require water to be sprayed onto foliage within their environment; geckos are an example. Tortoises and some snakes like to bathe in shallow bowls; this can aid in the uptake of water, and stimulates excretion. This method is an ideal way of administering supplements. If glucose-based supplements are dissolved in the water, the animal must be thoroughly washed after bathing to ensure that all the glucose has been removed from the skin, as this can encourage bacterial or fungal growth. Daily parenteral doses of water for rehydration are 10–25 ml/kg BW. In cases where nutritional support has been utilized, additional water at a rate of 1 ml per kilocalorie of energy provided should be administered.[2] Methods to increase water consumption in reptiles are described in Appendix 4.

Vertebrate prey

The feeding of live vertebrate prey is illegal in the UK. In countries where it is legal, it is not recommended. Reptiles can suffer serious injuries from live prey, especially from rodents. Prey that have been frozen for short periods of time are nutritionally equal to live prey. The nutrient value of the prey is dependent on their age and health. Obese prey contain over 50% fat, and therefore nutrient content relative to calories is decreased.[2] Care should also be taken that the prey do not carry any parasites or pathogenic organisms.

Invertebrate prey

Commercial prey such as crickets and mealworms are readily available, and many species thrive on these diets. When advising owners on the correct diet for their animals, careful research should be undertaken, and advice sought from reptile experts. The feeding of invertebrate prey is dependent on many factors, including the size of the prey and the species of the prey. Some lizards will base their diet around specific species of invertebrates.[2] A variety of appropriately sized invertebrates should be offered, including snails, slugs, moths, flies and other soft-bodied insects and non-venomous spiders.[2] Snails can prove an excellent calcium source, owing to the shell, which contains 28.3% calcium dry matter base (DMB).[2] Earthworms are often accepted by carnivorous and omnivorous reptiles that would naturally inhabit woodland.[2]

Plants

When offering vegetables to reptiles, the proportion of greens, fruit and vegetables differ between species. Reptiles from more arid environments will prefer to consume drier foods such as hay. Those from temperate or tropical habitats will prefer moist, sweet foods. Some species, such as tortoises, seem to prefer foods that are red, yellow or orange in colour. Hence, they tend to consume strawberries, apples, oranges, sweet potatoes and mangos readily.[2]

In cases of calcium deficiency, plants with high levels of oxalates should be avoided, as the oxalates bind the calcium and inhibit its absorption. Examples of plants high in oxalate levels include spinach, rhubarb, cabbage, peas and potatoes. Hypothyroidism can be induced if large quantities of plant material containing goitrogens are consumed, alongside a marginal iodine intake. Plants that contain large quantities of goitrogens include cabbage, kale, and other cruciferous plants. This stresses the importance of feeding a variety of different plants (grasses, fruits and vegetables) to reptiles (Box 20.1).

Fibre

Fibre provides calories through hindgut fermentation in herbivores, and is important in gut motility. Its role in exotic nutrition should not be underestimated. Excessive fibre, however, limits calorie intake and inhibits trace mineral absorption.[2]

Box 20.1 A typical tortoise diet for Mediterranean tortoises[4]

20% mixed green vegetables – cabbage, lettuce, spring greens

10% varied fruits – peach, pear, melon, tomato, mango, apple

45% coarse weeds and grasses

5% added mineral/vitamin supplement + extra calcium lactate

Feeding diets designed for non-reptilian species

Canine and feline diets are commonly fed to reptiles. The difference in nutrient demands between the species is not huge and reptiles can be fed these diets. Omnivores should be fed a low-fat product formulated for canine maintenance, whereas carnivores would require a high-protein diet formulated for cats. There is anecdotal evidence that the feeding of these diets long term can result in growth deformities in some species.[3] This may be due, in part, to these diets being overfed, and making up too high a proportion of the animal's total diet. Herbivore diets, such as pellets or hay cakes, can be safely fed to herbivorous reptiles, but again should only be a small proportion of the animal's total diet.

Supplements

Dusting of supplements onto food is recommended, as it seems to help prevent vitamin and mineral (especially calcium) deficiencies in insectivorous reptiles. It should, however, be applied with care and its limitations appreciated. Invertebrates contain little calcium, except for earthworms that ingest calcium-rich soil, and snail shells. The use of alfalfa has become widely recognized as a good protein and calcium source for herbivores.[2]

Care should be given to the route of supplement administration, as it can reduce the palatability of the diet; some nutrients can decompose more quickly if dissolved in water, and in some cases invertebrates can clean off any supplement used to dust them.

Commonly encountered malnutritions

Hypovitaminosis and hypervitaminosis A

Vitamin A deficiency is primarily noted in chelonians, but has also been reported in iguanas. Clinical symptoms of hypovitaminosis A include blepharoedema alongside, in chronic cases, solid whitish-yellow cellular debris underneath the eyelids.[2] Other symptoms include lethargy, anorexia and weight loss. In order to confirm hypovitaminosis A, a full thorough clinical and dietary history should be made. Blepharoedema can be caused through trauma, foreign bodies, pollen, and mycotic, bacterial or nematode infections.[2] Treatment of hypovitaminosis A is made through subcutaneous injections of 1500–2000 IU of parenteral vitamin A/kg BW. In mild cases this will need to be repeated once a week for 2 weeks; in more severe cases a longer period is required, often up to 6 weeks. Care must be given not to over-administrate, as hypervitaminosis can easily occur. Long-term preventative treatment should also be addressed in these cases, and mainly includes the involvement of foods rich in beta-carotene in the diet. These foods include dark leafy greens such as spinach, dandelions and broccoli; and orange-coloured vegetables such as butternut squash, carrots and sweet potatoes. Whole mice and fish are also good nutrient sources. Commercial diets and supplements can also provide required levels of the vitamin.

Hypervitaminosis A is also common in reptiles, as in mammals. The fat-soluble vitamin can easily be overdosed with the use of supplements and feeding of higher-fat diets. Supplementing vitamin A should only be recommended when a deficiency has been diagnosed. The use of a well-balanced diet should remove the need for these supplements.

Thiamin and vitamin E deficiencies

A common deficiency in aquatic carnivorous reptiles is deficiency of thiamin due to the high levels of thiaminases present in fish. Deficiencies in vitamin E can also be present, because of the high levels of polyunsaturated fatty acids. Fish with any sign of rancidity should not be fed, as this will indicate depletion in vitamin E levels. Thiamin deficiencies can be treated through oral or parenteral administration of dosages of 25 mg/kg BW.[2]

Protein deficiency

The prevalence of protein deficiency in reptiles is not well known. Animals that have a reduced food intake, poor diet or other poor husbandry factors can have a reduced protein intake. Animals that are fed whole prey can also suffer from these deficiencies if the animal is obese, because of a proportionate decrease in protein to fat percentages. Required levels of dietary proteins differ, depending on the animal's nutritional group, and are displayed in Table 20.2.

Metabolic bone disorder (MBD)

MBD is also known as fibrous oesteodystrophy or nutritional secondary hyperparathyroidism. MBD affecting reptiles is generally a chronic result of a deficiency of calcium or vitamin D, negative calcium to phosphorus ratio, and/or lack of exposure to ultraviolet (UV) light.

Ultraviolet light plays a necessary role in the synthesis of vitamin D_3 (1,25-dihydroxycholecalciferol). It should be noted that only UVB (wavelength range of 290–315 nm) will enable the process, and therefore it is vital that the UV lights used in reptile/chelonian vivariums cover both UVA and UVB spectra.[5] UV light is also necessary for the animal to achieve its POTZ for a proportion of the day, in order to activate the enzymes necessary for the synthesis of vitamin D_3. Window glass filters out UV rays and, therefore, sunshine through a window is of no value. Artificial light sources cannot replace natural sunlight, and it has been shown that those animals that have access to the natural light in an outdoor enclosure live longer, have better, healthier lives and grow bigger (Fig. 20.1). It should be remembered that renal disease can also cause MBD, and with some cases not being presented until later on in the disease/disorder process, it is sometimes difficult to differentiate the primary cause.

Levels of calcium should be monitored; on blood sampling both serum calcium and ionized calcium levels should be examined.

Gout

Gout can present in many forms; these include visceral, articular and periarticular, and can be either primary or secondary. Primary gout is due to an overproduction of uric acid, possibly related to enzyme defects. Secondary gout occurs when the

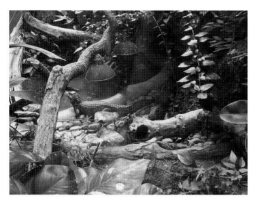

Figure 20.1 Environment and diet can be as varied as the species size.

hyperuricaemia results from an acquired chronic disease or drug that interferes with the normal balance between production and excretion of uric acid.[6] Diets excessive in protein can lead to a build-up of the primary nitrogenous metabolic product, uric acid. Uric acid is produced by the liver and excreted by the renal tubules. In mammals this process is achieved by filtration. Renal failure is common in reptiles, and when uric acid levels reach saturation point in the blood, it will crystallize out into the mucous membranes, pericardial sac, myocardium, liver and kidneys. Various risk factors will contribute towards the development of gout. These include renal damage, dehydration and an excessive intake of purine-rich meals. Cat food is high in purines, and gout often presents in animals fed a diet too high in animal protein.

Very little research has been conducted into the treatment of gout in reptiles, especially concerning medications. Prevention is better than cure, and owner education can never be initiated early enough. Husbandry and diet relating to the species of reptile being kept are the main points.

Diarrhoea

Diarrhoea can be defined as acute or chronic, as in mammals, though differences between small and large intestinal diarrhoea are not as commonly observed. Acute cases can be self-limiting, and be associated with vomiting. Causes of diarrhoea are similar to those in mammals, but husbandry plays a larger role. Feeding an animal at its incorrect temperature, or a meal that is too large can also have

an effect on the GIT system. Causes of diarrhoea include parasites, sudden change of diet, foreign bodies (if the animal is still feeding), viral infections, medications and the use of inappropriate foods.

Treatments of diarrhoea revolve around the initial cause. Any husbandry-related causes need to be addressed, and any parasites treated with the use of an appropriate parasiticide. Bacterial and fungal infections will require antimicrobial treatments.

Anorexia

Anorexia is a common clinical symptom of a number of different diseases or disorders. Treatment of the anorexia must include treatment, if possible, of the underlying cause. Anorexia can also be part of the animal's normal behaviour prior to hibernation. With any reptile being presented with anorexia it is vital to take a full dietary and husbandry history. Animals being fed the incorrect type of food, or at the wrong time, at the animal's wrong POTZ can all induce anorexia. In cases where husbandry is the causal problem, client education is required and client handouts or care sheets should be made use of. Recommendations to internet websites are also useful. Where more than one animal is housed together, feeding separately is encouraged, as a dominant individual may inhibit a subordinate from feeding.[2]

Once all husbandry aspects have been addressed, if anorexia still persists, nutritional support should be initiated.

Nutritional support

Nutritional support is often under-utilized in many veterinary practices, mainly due to the lack of the various different husbandry-related equipment required by reptiles. Nutritional support should only be instigated when the correct environmental conditions for the animal can also be achieved (Fig. 20.2). This includes gradients of temperature, humidity, UV light, delivery of water, provision of substrate, hiding places and cage furniture.[2]

The provision of water to all patients is vital, and in many cases requiring nutritional support, increased water consumption is required. Methods of encouraging patients to consume more water are covered in Appendix 4. Parenteral fluid therapy should always be utilized if required. Medications

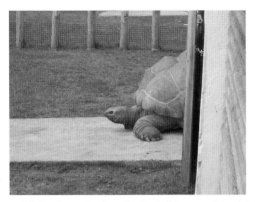

Figure 20.2 Good husbandry is vital for good health in all exotic species.

and supplements can also be administered via the water. If they are distasteful, and water consumption reduces, then alternative methods of administration are required.

Involuntary feeding can be managed by force-feeding, with the use of syringe feeding or stomach tubing. These processes can be very stressful for the animal, and can exacerbate any aversions towards food. 'Slap feeding' of carnivores can be used; this involves gently tapping the prey alongside the mouth of the carnivore. It is recommended that the prey be held in tongs when performing this task.

Post-hibernation problems

Common species of tortoises in the UK undergo hibernation. These species are *Testudo graeca* ('spur-thighed' or 'common' tortoise), *T. hermanni* (Hermann's tortoise) and *T. marginata* (marginated or margined tortoise). Hibernation should reflect what these species of tortoise would undertake in the wild. The length of hibernation should be no longer than 10–12 weeks. The correct diet for tortoises that undergo hibernation is exceptionally important, and an incorrect diet can result in serious problems, especially in respect to liver and kidney function. Sick or underweight tortoises should never be hibernated.

All tortoises should be clinically examined prior to hibernation and have anthelmintics administered. Vitamin injections are not recommended, and can cause abscesses. Prior to hibernation the tortoise will reduce its food intake; hibernation whilst there is still undigested food within the GIT is dangerous, and leads to many deaths each year. This is due to the undigested food decaying and producing large quantities of gas that can lead to tympanitic colic, and thus asphyxiation due to internal pressure on the tortoise's lungs.[4] Water consumption should be encouraged prior to hibernation, with the tortoise being placed in its hibernation accommodation with its bladder full of water. Placing a tortoise on a piece of absorbent paper will identify if it has urinated during the hibernation period. If it does, the tortoise must be woken up early, and placed under a heat lamp for the remainder of the winter. Hibernating tortoises will lose 1% of their bodyweight each month; weighing of the tortoise during this period is recommended, and can do no harm to the animal. Urinating during hibernation in a tortoise that is not woken up can result in renal failure, due to prolonged dehydration. It has been proposed that water is recirculated from the bladder in order to ensure correct hydration of the tortoise during the period of hibernation.

When tortoises are woken up early or are 'over-wintered' it is vital that they are maintained at the correct temperature. Tortoises that are not maintained at this correct temperature will not wake up properly, and will not eat or drink. Radiant heat can be obtained by placing a basking lamp over the tortoises; this tends to be a 100 watt bulb 30 cm over the animals. The tortoise must have sufficient room to move away from the lamp when required. A low waking-up temperature is the most common cause of post-hibernation anorexia, but health problems should always be eliminated. It is advisable to send all tortoise owners hibernation guides/care sheets at least 6 weeks prior to hibernation, so that tortoise health can be maintained.

References

1. Ackerman N. Critical care nutrition for exotics. VNJ 2005; 20(4):14–16.
2. Donoghue S, Langenberg J. Nutrition. In: Mader DR, ed. Reptile medicine and surgery. Philadelphia: WB Saunders; 1996:148–174.
3. Tefend M, Berryhill SA. Companion animal clinical nutrition. In: McCurnin DM, Bassert JM, eds. Clinical textbook for veterinary technicians. 6th edn. St Louis, Missouri: Elsevier Saunders; 2006:438–492.
4. Highfield AC. Care sheet: safer hibernation and your tortoise. 2006. Online. Available:http://www.tortoisetrust.org
5. Heards D, Fleming G, Lock B, et al. Lizards. In: Redrobe S, Meredith A, eds. BSAVA manual of exotic pets. 4th edn. Gloucester: BSAVA Publications; 2002:223–240.
6. Mader DR. Gout. In: Mader DR, ed. Reptile medicine and surgery. Philadelphia: WB Saunders; 1996:374–379.

Appendices

Puppies and kittens

Why does my puppy eat its own faeces?
Puppies commonly practice coprophagia, and this can be due to attractive food residues in the faeces. The practice can also be acquired when house training a puppy. If the puppy is badly disciplined when it defecates in the house, it can start consuming the faeces in order to avoid being disciplined. Common practices in order to stop this behaviour include feeding the puppy pineapple, as it makes the faeces very distasteful, and sprinkling chilli powder on the faeces. In some cases where there is a lot of undigested material in the faeces, it is important to advise faecal analysis in order to establish any GIT abnormalities.

Can I give my puppy or kitten milk?
Once a puppy or kitten has been weaned from its mother, there is no nutritional reason to provide milk. The use of cow's or goat's milk is not advised as it contains higher levels of lactose than bitch's or queen's milk, and can trigger food intolerances. This also applies to commercially manufactured milk for cats. Some of these products even have a disclaimer on the packaging, warning of this problem.

Should I stick to breeder's dietary recommendations?
If the animal is on a good-quality, complete balanced diet that is suitable for that individual then there is no need to initiate a change. If the owner is unhappy about the diet, or the diet is not suitable, then a change should occur. Some owners worry that they do not wish to continue with the breeder's recommendation, but they should also remember that the pet now belongs to them, and it is their choice.

Can I feed my puppy bones?
Anyone working within the veterinary practice setting has seen the consequences of allowing dogs to eat bones – gut perforations, diarrhoea, etc. Puppies' teeth are also fairly weak in comparison to adult teeth, and can easily break. It is recommended that advice given to owners is that no bones should be fed to dogs.

How often should I feed my pup?
Feeding schedules of puppies should be based on the individual. Some small-breed puppies will have difficulty consuming more than a very small meal, because of limited stomach size, and therefore more frequent meals may be required. Frequency of feeding also depends on the age of the animal. When advising clients on their puppies' meal frequency these points should be conveyed, and a decision should be made around the answers. Some puppies will self-limit and free-choice feeding is suitable; some will benefit from three to four meals per day.

My large-breed puppy is 8 months old and overweight, which diet should it be on?
A full dietary history is required in these cases as excess weight could be due to too much of the diet being fed, treats, table scraps and training aids. Transferring the puppy onto an adult diet can help, but it should be remembered that the dog will need to consume more in order to have the correct energy intake, and this will mean an increase in calcium levels; excessive calcium could be consumed as a consequence. Reducing the

amount of puppy food being fed, and the removal of any other foods, should be encouraged, alongside increased exercise levels.

Can I feed my pet a raw meat and bone diet?
There is a common trend towards feeding dogs in this manner, in order to mirror what an undomesticated dog would consume in the wild. Raw meat and bones do not do this, as dogs scavenge, and also consume the skin, hair and other soft tissues of their prey. Bones can also be detrimental to GIT health, and uncooked meats can contain harmful bacteria. The domesticate dogs of today have lost some of their natural immunity, and can therefore have GIT upsets on this diet.

Rabbits

Can I give my rabbits treats?
There are many treats designed for rabbits on the market. Many have a high simple sugar content (i.e. chocolate-flavoured or yoghurt drops) and should be avoided as they can contribute towards obesity. Treats that can be recommended include hay cakes and vegetables.

What vegetables can I safely give my rabbit?
Recommended vegetables are those that are not too high in simple sugars or minerals. Carrot tops are a favourite (owners can be confused by this and it should be conveyed that the green tops are the most beneficial part of the vegetable), as are broccoli and kale. Lettuce and cucumbers have a very high water content and contain negligible amounts of fibre, and can contribute towards diarrhoea.

How much should I be feeding my rabbit?
The diets of rabbits should be made up of 95–100% hay, grass and vegetables. If a concentrate is to be fed, then an average-sized rabbit should receive a couple of tablespoonfuls daily.

Equines

Do I have to feed my horse concentrates?
If your horse is a good doer, and maintains its weight, BCS and MCS without the need for concentrates, then there is no requirement to feed it hard feeds. Animals that require concentrates are those that require extra nutrients because their energy expenditure is greater than what they can consume from hay and grass.

My horse eats and licks at the soil; does it have a mineral deficiency?
Some horses do lick and eat soil purely due to the taste. Some soils have high iron content, and some horses like the taste of it. In some cases, however, a mineral deficiency could be present.

Dietary changes

Why does my animal have diarrhoea when it changes diet?
Changes in diet can cause transient diarrhoea. This can be due to the microbial population in the GIT having to adapt to the new nutrient make-up of the new diet. Any dietary changes should be slow so that the microbial populations can adapt over a period of time in order to accommodate the changes. The GIT metabolic physiology also has to adapt to the new nutrient differences.

How do I get my pet to change its diet?
Some animals, no matter how slowly you perform a transitional change, will not want to consume a new diet. In some cases changing to an intermediate diet can benefit (i.e. instead of changing directly to a very restricted salt diet, changing initially to a slightly less restricted salt diet as an intermediate step can help). Adding a very highly palatable diet to the new diet, and then slowly reducing this once the animal has accepted the new diet can also help. In some cases when changing the texture of the diet, transition can be very difficult. Animals are exceptionally adept at eating around the desired kibble, and picking out only the bits that they want. In some exceptionally difficult cases, the use of a blender has been very helpful. The animal is then unable to pick out the bits it wants, and has to consume the whole mixture. Altering the percentages of old and new diet will encourage the animal to move onto the new diet, and accustom it to the new taste. Once this has been achieved, blending the food less and less

will increase the particle sizes until the animal is eating the diet as it comes out of the packaging.

Which diet do you recommend?
This is a very common question, and to make a recommendation you must wholly support it, and be able to tell the owner why. In some circumstances some owners may not be able to afford what you recommend, or the animal may not like the diet. In these cases it can be useful to have an A list and a B list. The A list contains first-choice recommendations and premium diets. The B list tends to contain second-choice diets and possibly supermarket diets.

Exercising

Why does my dog or horse always defecate when exercising?
Moderate exercising and movement encourage defecation by increasing peristalsis, another reason why movement is encouraged in horses with colic. When intense exercising occurs, the blood supply to the digestive system is reduced, hence the recommendation not to exercise after a meal.

How long should I give after feeding before exercising?
This does depend heavily on the nutrient content of the diet. High-fat diets will take longer to leave the stomach than carbohydrate diets. It is recommended that at least 1 hour be left before exercising.

Is it true that you should withhold food and large amounts of water post-exercising?
The consumption of large amounts of food and water after exercising should be avoided, until the animal's body has returned to its resting status. Water can be offered, but in small quantities.

Clinical nutrition

If my pet is suffering from more than one specific problem, which takes precedence?
If more than one specific problem exists, then the most potentially serious disease should come first.

In some cases a compromise can be met, and use should be made of the manufacturer's help lines.

Should my epileptic pet be on a protein-restricted diet?
There has been some anecdotal evidence that protein-restricted diets aid in controlling seizures in human epileptic sufferers. There has also been evidence that high-protein, high-fat diets can also aid in controlling seizures. As of yet, no scientific studies have been conducted on animals concerning dietary protein levels and epilepsy.

Should my epileptic pet be on a salt-restricted diet?
Animals that are receiving potassium bromide as part of their medications can benefit from a lower-salt diet. This is due to the dietary salt binding with the potassium bromide, lowering its efficiency.

My pet is on medications, and has been recommended a high-fibre diet; won't the fibre content affect the medication?
Some medications can be bound up by dietary fibre. In these cases it is advisable to administer the medication at a different time from that of feeding.

Can I feed my diabetic dog treats?
Diabetic animals can receive treats, but it does depend on the treat. Treats that are high in simple sugars must be avoided, as should treats that are low in fat. Low-fat foods tend to have a higher sugar level. If a treat is to be fed, i.e. between meals because the dog is slightly hungry, then it should be given each day, and the same amount given. It is best to avoid additional foodstuffs, but if the animal does appear to be slightly low then it can be beneficial. If an owner is complaining of this, a glucose curve should be initiated in order to identify if the animal is receiving too much insulin.

Which dental treat/diet should I use, and can it be used in combination with my pet's normal diet?
Some dental diets are complete diets, and can be fed on their own, and are most beneficial when fed in this manner. Some are complementary and are designed to make up only a proportion of the

daily diet. In these cases it is important to recalculate the quantity of other foods that make up the diet. Guidance can be gained from the manufacturers on the minimum percentage that can be fed and still have a beneficial effect.

What should I do when the animal doesn't lose weight?

All animals are individuals, and some will lose weight very easily, whereas others will find losing weight exceptionally difficult. If an animal is not losing weight in the manner that it should be, it is important to re-ask to confirm that the animal is not receiving any table scraps, treats, etc., and that the animal is only receiving the calculated quantity of diet. If everything checks out, then a 10% reduction of the diet should be made. If the owner is not willing to do this because the animal is starting to scavenge, then suggest a 10% increase in exercise levels. If the animal is on a weight-reduction diet based around a low fat level, then changing to a low-energy and high-fibre diet can be very beneficial, as it will help to make the animal feel fuller.

What treats can I feed my overweight pet?

Obese animals tend to be obese due to the excessive consumption of food, mainly treats. Telling owners that they cannot feed treats can be very difficult. Some owners feel that their bond with their pet is reinforced with the giving and receiving of treats. Some manufacturers do specifically make treats that can be used alongside an obesity diet, each treat having a known calorie value, and will advise on the quantity of diet that should be removed from the daily quota. In some animals simply giving them one or two kibbles of the weight reduction diet can be the same as giving a treat. It is advisable that the owner weighs out the required daily quota in the morning. Any food that the animal receives needs to come out of this pre-measured amount.

When using a food trial, can I give my animal treats of the same flavours?

In most cases the answer is no. Some commercially manufactured treats contain different additives, colourants and ingredients. So even if the animal is on a lamb and rice only diet, the giving of treats that are also lamb and rice can be detrimental. In some cases, however, some manufacturers also make treats that can be used alongside diets utilized in food trials. If advising a pet owner on this, the use of the kibble as a treat, as in obesity/weight management programmes, is the best method.

Exotics

Can I feed my tortoise cat/dog food?

This is highly dependent on the species of tortoise. Tortoises that are herbivores do not require animal protein in their diet. Those that are omnivores can benefit from a very small percentage of their daily nutrient requirements being obtained from cat or dog foods.

Should I be feeding vitamin and mineral supplements to my pet?

Tortoises can benefit from the addition of minerals to their diet; vitamin supplements should be used with caution because of the danger of over-supplementation. The requirements for vitamin and mineral supplements in all reptile diets are highly dependent on the quality of their food or prey.

Do I need to get a UV lamp and/or heat lamp for my tortoise if she lives outside?

This depends on the species of tortoise you have, and which country you live in. In the UK you will need these lamps, especially if you need to wake up your tortoise during hibernation.

I have been told that handling my tortoise during hibernation can harm it?

This is completely untrue. Regular weighing and inspection of your tortoise is required during the hibernation period, to ensure that it has not urinated, or lost excessive amounts of weight.

Appendix 2
Food conversions

Cats and dogs

The period of transition for transferring over to a new diet depends on the individual animal. Having detailed information which can be relayed to the owner is of importance, as an unsuccessful transition to a new diet can put the owner off the new diet completely, and the prospect of changing in the future.

When transferring from a lifestage diet to a prescription diet, longer transitional periods may also be required. This is dependent on the changes in the ratios of nutrients in the diet (protein, fat, fibre levels) and/or alterations in metabolism (diarrhoea, fat maldigestion).

Birds

Birds can be especially fastidious concerning changes in diet, and patience and persistence are required. The recommended diet for companion kept birds (e.g. parrots) is a complete balanced pelleted diet. Some will immediately convert to pellets but some take longer, especially those that are 'seed junkies'. In order to 'wean' the bird off its existing diet, a few days prior to attempting the conversion, reduce the amount of seed that is being fed, do not top-up any food that is already there. This will encourage the bird to eat the diet being offered, and not just pick out its favourite bits. On the day that conversion is to commence, offer the bird a small amount of its normal diet (whether it is seeds or pellets) and leave this in the cage for half an hour. This will ensure that the bird has received a meal. After half an hour remove this food and replace it with a small amount of the new diet; this will be left with the bird for the remainder of the day. Parrots are naturally inquisitive and will investigate the new diet; if the regular diet is left in the cage the parrot will be less likely to investigate the new diet, and to eat it. It is important to offer only a limited amount of the new diet, as a larger amount will encourage the bird to play with its food and rummage looking for its regular food, especially if it cannot see the bottom of the dish. For the evening meal, it is always recommended to give the bird fresh fruit and vegetables (even when feeding a completed pelleted diet). If the bird will not eat fruit and vegetables, the original diet should be offered. This way you are sure that the bird has had an evening meal.

The following day repeat the same pattern, but leave the original diet in the cage for a shorter time, approximately 20–25 minutes. Each day, reduce the amount of time that the bird has with the original diet in the morning, and increase the time that it has with the new diet during the day. Converting birds in this manner does take a lot of time and determination. Those birds that are addicted to high-fat seeds can be very stubborn, but the key is to be more determined than the bird. By offering fruit and vegetable you are ensuring that the bird will not starve. In some cases no matter how well you persist in the conversion, the bird does not acknowledge the pellets as food. Methods to combat this are serving the pellets in the same way as the original diet, encouraging copying by showing the bird someone or another bird consuming the pellets, or moistening the pellets with the bird's favourite fruit juice.

Rabbits and horses

Any changes in diet need to be made slowly, as in other species. The role of the hindgut fermenters make this even more important because of the changes in gut flora that will need to occur in order to digest the new diet. Rapid changes can lead to groups of bacteria that are no longer required dying off quickly. As this occurs, endotoxins can be released into the gut lumen and subsequently absorbed into the bloodstream. When changes in diet are made over a period of time, the normal flora populations adapt slowly, without releasing high levels of endotoxins.

Appendix 3

Diet history sheet

Animal's information

Animal's name:
Client name:
Current weight: Optimal weight: BCS:
Breed: Age: Sex: M/F N/E
Current diseases:
Medications:
Activity level of the animal:
Quantity of exercise the animal receives:
Appetite levels:

Dietary information

Current brand of food being fed:
Is the diet: moist/dry/mixed
                      complete/complementary
Quantities at each meal:
Number of meals:
Treats being fed, and quantity:
Table/human foods:
    Breakfast
    Lunch
    Dinner
    Between meals
Food covering medications:
Food additives:
Vitamins/supplements:
Palatable medications:

Owner and environmental information

How many pets are in the household?
Do they feed together?
Where is the pet fed?
Is there competition for food?
Does the animal have access to other pets'
      food (neighbour)?
Who feeds the animal?
Are there other people in the household?
Does the animal scavenge?
Is more than one animal fed out of each
      feeding dish?
Is the food measured out?

Appendix 4
Methods of increasing water consumption in animals

Increased quantities of water within the diet are required for certain clinical diseases or disorders. Encouraging an animal to increase its consumption of water can be difficult, and a number of different methods may be required in order to achieve sufficient quantities consumed.

Cats

Cats can be extremely fastidious in what, when and where they eat or drink. In order to increase water consumption, the availability of water needs to be increased. This can be achieved by placing more water bowls around the cat's environment (both inside and outside the house), using different types of water. Tap water that is chlorinated does smell, even more so to a cat. Allowing the water to stand for a period of time can remove a large portion of the chlorine and make it more palatable to the cat. Cats that live in a multi-cat household can find eating and drinking alongside other cats very intimidating. Making food and water available in a place where the particular cat feels safe can be of benefit. The water content of the diet should also be increased; this can involve changing the cat over to a moist diet, or adding water to a moist diet. Cats tend not to consume dry biscuits that have had water added to them.

Dogs

Encouraging dogs to drink more fluids can be easier in some cases than it is with cats. Along with increasing the availability of water to the dog, and allowing the water to stand for a period of time, the use of flavoured waters can tempt some dogs, but be careful of brands that are high in sugar. Ice cubes can also be used, and are especially useful in hot temperatures.

Horses

Because it is a prey species, it is important to ensure that the horse is not alarmed when trying to drink. Horses will resist drinking from containers that are narrow and deep, as they can obscure their vision of any potential predators. The use of soaked hay can dramatically increase water consumption in stable-kept horses, as can increasing the water content of hard feeds, and the use of soaked sugar beet.

Rabbits

Encouraging a rabbit to drink more fluids is very difficult, but can be achieved. Thought should be given to the type of water container that the rabbit drinks from, whether the rabbit prefers a bowl or water bottle. The use of grasses and hays that have either been soaked or are wet can be advantageous. Sprinkling the grass before putting the rabbit out can help increase water consumption.

Birds/reptiles

Watching these animals in the wild can demonstrate ideal ways of increasing water consumption in these species. Many birds and reptiles obtain fluids from rainfall dripping from leaves. Setting up a drip line that drips water onto foliage can actively encourage the animal to drink more. The use of rabbit/small animal water bottles has been shown to be extremely useful with birds, with parrots especially liking to use this method. Water can also be injected into whole prey in order to increase water consumption.

Appendix 5
Unit conversion tables

Mass (weight)

1 kilogram (kg)	=	2.204 lb (pounds)
1 ounce (oz, avoirdupois)	=	28.3 g (grams)
1 ounce (oz, troy)	=	31.1 g (grams)
1 pound (lb)	=	16 oz (ounces)
		454 g (grams)
1 stone	=	14 lb (pounds)
		6.35 kg (kilograms)
1 hundredweight (cwt)	=	112 lb (pounds)
		8 stones
		50.8 kg (kilograms)
1 ton (imperial or UK)	=	2240 lb (pounds)
		160 stones
		20 hundredweight (cwt)
		1016 kg (kilograms)
1 ton (short ton or US)	=	2000 lb (pounds)
		907 kg (kilograms)
1 tonne (metric)	=	2204 lb (pounds)

Volume

1 imperial fluid ounce (fl oz)	=	28.41 ml
1 imperial pint	=	20 fluid ounces (fl oz)
		0.568 litres
1 imperial quart	=	1.137 litres
1 imperial (UK) gallon	=	160 fluid ounces (fl oz)
		8 pints
		4 quarts
		4.546 litres
1 US fluid ounce (US fl oz)	=	29.6 ml
1 US pint	=	16 US fluid ounces (US fl oz)
		0.473 litres
1 US quart	=	0.946 litres
1 US gallon	=	128 US fluid ounces (US fl oz)
		8 US pints
		4 US quarts
		6.785 litres

Temperature

Celsius (°C) $°C = 5/9 (°F - 32)$	Fahrenheit (°F) $°F = 9/5 (°C) + 32$
−273.15	−459.67
−40	−40
−17.78	0
0	32
10	50
20	68
30	86
35	95
36.0	96.8
36.5	97.7
37.0	98.6
37.5	99.5
38.0	100.4
38.5	101.3
39.0	102.2
39.5	103.1
40.0	104.0
40.5	104.9
41.0	105.8
41.5	106.7
42.0	107.6
42.5	108.5
43.0	109.4
43.5	110.3
44.0	111.2
44.5	112.1
45.0	113.0
45.5	113.9
46.0	114.8
50	122
60	140

Celsius (°C) $°C = 5/9 (°F - 32)$	Fahrenheit (°F) $°F = 9/5 (°C) + 32$
70	158
80	176
90	194
100	212
150	302
200	392
300	572
400	752
500	932
600	1112
700	1292
800	1472
900	1652
1000	1832

Multiple choice questions

Anatomy and physiology

Q1. What is the dentition of a rabbit?
(a) $2 \times \{I2/1 : C0/0 : P3/2 : M3/3\}$.
(b) $2 \times \{I1/1 : C0/0 : P3/2 : M3/3\}$.
(c) $2 \times \{I1/1 : C0/0 : P3/3 : M3/3\}$.
(d) $2 \times \{I2/1 : C0/0 : P3/3 : M3/3\}$.

Q2. What is the correct order of the digestive system of the stomach?
(a) Pylorus, fundus, cardia.
(b) Cardia, fundus, pylorus.
(c) Fundus, pylorus, cardia.
(d) Fundus, cardia, pylorus.

Q3. How is a micelle involved in digestion?
(a) Aids in the diffusion of nutrients.
(b) Aids in the absorption of fats.
(c) Aids in breaking down fats.
(d) None of the above.

Q4. Pepsinogen is activated by what to produce pepsin?
(a) Gastrin.
(b) Alkaline environment in the small intestine.
(c) Hydrochloric acid in the stomach.
(d) Lipase.

Q5. The teeth of equines are:
(a) Aradicular hypsodont.
(b) Brachyodont.
(c) Continuously erupting throughout life.
(d) Radicular hypsodont.

Q6. Which enzyme is present in the saliva of dogs?
(a) Lipase.
(b) Ptyalin.
(c) Lactase.
(d) Saliva of dogs does not contain any enzymes.

Q7. Active transport involves the use of:
(a) Water.
(b) Sodium.
(c) Potassium.
(d) Energy in the form of ATP.

Q8. The salivary glands of the dog and cat include:
(a) Zygomatic, sublingual, mandibular and parotid.
(b) Zygomatic, hyoid, mandibular and parotid.
(c) Hyoid, mandibular and parotid.
(d) Hyoid, mandibular, zygomatic.

Q9. The order of the three sections of the large intestine is:
(a) Descending, transverse, ascending.
(b) Transverse, descending, ascending.
(c) Ascending, transverse, descending.
(d) Ascending, descending, transverse.

Q10. Plant material is digested in the caecum in horses and rabbits into:
(a) Starch.
(b) Short-chain fatty acids.
(c) Water.
(d) Polysaccharides.

Nutrients

Q1. How many essential amino acids does the dog require?
(a) 11.
(b) 10.
(c) 9.
(d) 13.

Q2. Which essential fatty acids are required in the diet of the cat?
(a) Linoleic, linolenic and arachidonic.
(b) Lipoproteins, arachidonic, linolenic.
(c) Lipoproteins, arachidonic, linoleic.
(d) Phospholipids, arachidonic, linolenic.

Q3. How many kcal are provided by 1 gram of fat?
(a) 4.
(b) 9.
(c) 3.5.
(d) 2.5.

Q4. Which nutrient will provide the most energy per gram?
(a) Fibre.
(b) Fat.
(c) Carbohydrate.
(d) Protein.

Q5. Which nutrient cannot be digested by mammalian enzymes within the digestive system?
(a) Cellulose.
(b) Protein.
(c) Simple carbohydrates.
(d) Soluble carbohydrates.

Q6. The main function of vitamin E is?
(a) Formation of prothrombin.
(b) Aiding in tooth formation.
(c) As an antioxidant.
(d) Aiding in absorption of calcium from the gut.

Q7. Free radicals are:
(a) By-products of chemical reactions.
(b) A type of vitamin.
(c) Both (a) and (d).
(d) Highly reactive and unstable molecules.

Q8. What is a prebiotic?
(a) Nutrients given by mouth to manipulate the gut flora populations.
(b) Populations of microorganisms given by mouth.
(c) Yeast.
(d) None of the above.

Q9. Which are the fat-soluble vitamins?
(a) A, D, E and K.
(b) A, D and E.
(c) A, C, E and K.
(d) D, E and K.

Q10. A function of iodine in the body is:
(a) To aid in bone development.
(b) As a component of the growth hormone thyroxine.
(c) As a component of connective tissue.
(d) To aid in a healthy immune system.

Feeding calculations

Q1. What is one of the correct equations for calculating RER?
(a) $(70 \times$ Weight in kg$) + 30$ kcal.
(b) $(30 \times$ Weight in kg$) + 30$ kcal.
(c) $(30 \times$ Weight in g$) + 70$ kcal.
(d) $(30 \times$ Weight in kg$) + 70$ kcal.

Q2. What is the RER of a 15-kg dog?
(a) 520 kcal.
(b) 1080 kcal.
(c) 480 kcal.
(d) 45030 kcal.

Q3. What is the MER of a 7.5-kg dog, in moderate exercise, assuming a factor rate of 2?
(a) 1110 kcal.
(b) 510 kcal.
(c) 590 kcal.
(d) 45014 kcal.

Q4. *A dog requires 600 kcal per day. How much of a diet containing 133 kcal/100 g of ME as fed requires to be fed?*
(a) 451 g.
(b) 45 g.
(c) 800 g.
(d) 250 g.

Q5. *A pet food is 70% water, and on an as-fed basis it contains 10% fat. What percentage would this equate to on a dry-matter basis?*
(a) 10%.
(b) 50%.
(c) 33.3%.
(d) 25%.

Q6. *A diet contains 86 mg of sodium per 100 g of food. If the diet has an energy density of 300 kcal/100 g as fed, how much sodium will there be in 100 kcal ME?*
(a) 28.67 mg.
(b) 2.86 mg.
(c) 258 mg.
(d) 28.67 g.

Q7. *A diet contains 84 mg of potassium per 50 g of food. How much of the diet would have to be fed for the animal to gain 420 mg of potassium?*
(a) 10 g.
(b) 705.6 g.
(c) 500 g.
(d) 250 g.

Q8. *If a diet contains 2.2 g of potassium citrate per kg of diet, how much would a dog receive if it were fed 305 g of food per day?*
(a) 67.1 mg.
(b) 0.671 g.
(c) 6.71 g.
(d) 6.71 mg.

Q9. *If a diet contained 394 kcal for each can of diet fed, how many calories would a cat receive if it ate two-thirds of a can per day?*
(a) 131 kcal.
(b) 200 kcal.
(c) 262.6 kcal.
(d) 150 kcal.

Q10. *An overweight dog currently receives 225 g of food per day. You need to reduce the amount by 10%, as it is not losing weight. How much per day does it need to be fed?*
(a) 200 g.
(b) 150 g.
(c) 215 g.
(d) 202.5 g.

Food and feeding

Q1. *A complementary diet is one that:*
(a) Should make up 100% of the animal's diet.
(b) Could be fed as a treat alongside a complete diet.
(c) Should be fed in combination with other diets to make a balanced diet.
(d) Both (b) and (c).

Q2. *An example of a humectant is:*
(a) Propylene glycol.
(b) Glucose syrup.
(c) Glycerine.
(d) All of the above.

Q3. *Palatability of a diet can be affected by:*
(a) Clinical illness of the animal.
(b) Texture and odour.
(c) Fat, protein and salt levels.
(d) All of the above.

Q4. *Which of the following must be declared on a pet food label?*
(a) Name and address of the manufacturer.
(b) Percentage of carbohydrate present.
(c) Vitamin B levels (if added).
(d) None of the above.

Q5. *When must water content be included on the pet food label?*
(a) When it exceeds 20% of the dietary content.
(b) When it exceeds 14% of the dietary content.
(c) It never needs to be included.
(d) When it is under 14% of the dietary content.

Q6. Seafood/fish ingredients in cat foods:
(a) Are often used to appeal to owners.
(b) Should not be used.
(c) Can cause heavy metal poisonings.
(d) Both (b) and (c).

Q7. Transition of animals from one food to another:
(a) Should be done abruptly.
(b) Should occur over a minimum of 7 days.
(c) Can be achieved by wetting down the diet.
(d) Should occur by placing the new diet down and leaving it until eaten.

Q8. What is the most important characteristic of a diet?
(a) A diet that appeals to the owner.
(b) Appealing shapes and colours.
(c) Optimal nutrient profile for the individual's lifestage.
(d) The packaging.

Q9. Time-restricted feeding is:
(a) When an unlimited quantity of diet is offered for a set period of time.
(b) When a set volume of diet is offered for a set period of time.
(c) Either (a) or (b).
(d) None of the above.

Q10. Different kibble shapes in dry diets:
(a) Are used to appeal to owners.
(b) Can be beneficial to specific breeds.
(c) When coupled with colour have a higher palatability.
(d) Both (a) and (b).

Lifestage diets

Q1. What is the optimal calcium : phosphorus ratio for growing large-breed dogs?
(a) 1 : 1 to 1.5 : 1.
(b) 1 : 2.
(c) 2 : 1.
(d) 1 : 1 to 1 : 2.

Q2. When does peak lactation commonly occur in the bitch?
(a) 1 week post-parturition.
(b) 3–4 weeks post-parturition.
(c) 1 week pre-parturition.
(d) At time of parturition.

Q3. Senior animals benefit from a diet:
(a) Low in protein but high in fibre.
(b) Low in fibre, high in fat.
(c) Restricted protein, lower in salts.
(d) High in salt in order to increase palatability.

Q4. Pregnant queens should have their diet increased:
(a) At the start of the pregnancy.
(b) During the second half of gestation.
(c) During the last 2 weeks of gestation.
(d) Queens do not require an increase in energy levels.

Q5. Pregnant bitches should have their diet increased:
(a) Bitches do not require an increase in energy levels.
(b) From the start of the pregnancy.
(c) During the last 2 weeks of gestation.
(d) After the first 4–5 weeks of gestation.

Q6. How often should an adult dog be fed?
(a) Once a day.
(b) Totally dependent on the individual animal.
(c) Every other day.
(d) Ad libitum feeding should be utilized.

Q7. A lactating Great Dane should be fed:
(a) A large-breed puppy diet.
(b) Large-breed maintenance diet.
(c) A puppy diet aimed at small to medium breeds.
(d) Either (a) or (c).

Q8. 'Light' diets are aimed at:
(a) Animals that need to lose weight.
(b) Animals predisposed to putting on weight.

(c) Older animals.

(d) Either (a) or (b).

Q9. *Neonate foals often practice copraphagia:*

(a) In order to populate their intestines with microflora from the dam.

(b) Because of lack of nutrition.

(c) Because of poor husbandry.

(d) None of the above.

Q10. *Oils are commonly added to equine diets in order to:*

(a) Provide an energy source higher in calories than proteins and carbohydrates.

(b) Aid in palatability.

(c) Help give the horse a glossy coat.

(d) All of the above.

Clinical nutrition

Q1. *What is an alternative name for yellow fat disease?*

(a) Pansteatitis.

(b) Pancreatitis.

(c) Obesity.

(d) Pollakiuria.

Q2. *Clinical nutritional aims for a cat suffering from CRF include?*

(a) Increase weight of the animal.

(b) Aid in reducing clinical symptoms.

(c) Improve quality of life for the animal.

(d) All of the above.

Q3. *The use of glycoaminoglycans is advocated in:*

(a) Cystitis.

(b) Arthritis.

(c) FLUTD.

(d) All of the above.

Q4. *For the dissolution of struvite (triple phosphate) crystals, the urine is required to be:*

(a) Alkaline (pH 9–11).

(b) Acidic (pH 5.9–6.1).

(c) Acidic (pH 3–4).

(d) Alkaline (pH 7–8).

Q5. *Which mineral levels should be controlled in diets aimed at cats with oxalate uroliths?*

(a) Potassium.

(b) Phosphorus.

(c) Magnesium.

(d) Calcium.

Q6. L-*Carnitine is often supplemented in diets in order to:*

(a) Reduce workload on the liver and kidneys.

(b) Help maintain lean body mass.

(c) Help improve fat metabolism.

(d) Both (b) and (c).

Q7. *The diet of choice for an overweight diabetic dog would be:*

(a) High fibre, low carbohydrate.

(b) High carbohydrate, low fat.

(c) Low fat.

(d) Low protein, high carbohydrate.

Q8. *The ideal diet for a critically ill or convalescent patient would be:*

(a) High carbohydrate, high fibre.

(b) High fibre, low fat.

(c) High protein, high fat.

(d) High in vitamins and minerals.

Q9. *Colitis can be treated with:*

(a) A diet high in fibre.

(b) A highly digestible diet.

(c) A hypoallergenic diet.

(d) All of the above.

Q10. *Poor dentition in the rabbit can be attributed to:*

(a) Genetics.

(b) Poor diet.

(c) Reduced access to chewing behaviours.

(d) All of the above.

Q11. *Weight reduction can be achieved through:*

(a) Reduction in calorific intake.

(b) Increased exercise regimen.

(c) Dietary supplements.

(d) All of the above.

Q12. *The restriction of which mineral has been shown to slow the progression of renal disease?*
(a) Potassium.
(b) Calcium.
(c) Phosphorus.
(d) Magnesium.

Q13. *When an animal presents with more than one clinical disease that can be aided by a nutritional diet, what should you do?*
(a) Mix the two diets together.
(b) Feed for the most serious of the diseases/disorders.
(c) Gain advice from the manufacturers of the diet.
(d) Both (b) and (c).

Q14. *B vitamins are commonly supplemented in clinical diets because:*
(a) They are commonly lost when polyuria is present.
(b) During illness, the B complex vitamins are metabolized faster.
(c) They are not supplemented.
(d) Both (a) and (b).

Q15. *Taurine supplementation in cardiac diets occurs:*
(a) Only in canine diets.
(b) Only in feline diets.
(c) Never.
(d) In both (a) and (b).

Q16. *Antioxidant supplementation is recommended in animals suffering from:*
(a) Arthritis.
(b) Liver disease.
(c) Cancer.
(d) All of the above.

Q17. *Supplementary enzymes of amylase and lipase should be used in cases of:*
(a) Pancreatitis.
(b) Exocrine pancreatic insufficiency.
(c) Diabetes.
(d) Both (a) and (b).

Q18. *When an animal is suffering from constipation or faecal impaction:*
(a) A high-fibre diet must be fed to remove the impaction.
(b) Treatment (medical or surgical) to remove the impaction should be used.
(c) Both (a) and (b).
(d) A high-protein diet should be fed.

Q19. *During recovery from surgery, food should be offered:*
(a) Straight away.
(b) Once the animal has recovered sufficiently.
(c) At a time dependent on the surgery performed.
(d) Both (b) and (c).

Q20. *An increased water consumption can be beneficial in cases of:*
(a) FLUTD.
(b) Diabetes.
(c) EPI.
(d) CRF.

Exotic nutrition

Q1. *Over-consumption of raw unsupplemented fish can result in:*
(a) Niacin deficiency.
(b) Vitamin C deficiency.
(c) Thiamin deficiency.
(d) Vitamin D deficiency.

Q2. *Sunflower seeds should not be fed to birds as:*
(a) They contain addictive chemicals.
(b) They are high in fat, and have limited other nutrients.
(c) They can be fed to birds, just not African Greys.
(d) They directly cause gout.

Q3. *Hypocalcaemia in parrots can be treated with:*
(a) Use of a UV light.
(b) Supplementation with calcium.
(c) Supplementation with vitamin D_3.
(d) All of the above.

Q4. *Which nutrients tend to be deficient in seeds?*
   (a) Omega fatty acids.
   (b) Vitamin A.
   (c) Essential amino acids.
   (d) All of the above.

Q5. *Dusting of invertebrates should occur, but has limitations because:*
   (a) Most of the supplement can be removed or fall off.
   (b) The supplement can reduce the palatability of the prey.
   (c) Supplements are not nutritionally balanced.
   (d) Both (a) and (b).

Q6. *Hypervitaminosis A is commonly seen in reptiles because of:*
   (a) Over-supplementation of the vitamin.
   (b) Being fed cat food.
   (c) Being fed dog food.
   (d) Being fed vegetables.

Q7. *If a hibernating tortoise wakes up early from hibernation, what should be recommended?*
   (a) Placing it back into its box in order to continue hibernation.
   (b) Warming it up, and actively encouraging it to eat and drink.
   (c) Leaving it alone; it will either stay awake or go back to hibernation as it wishes.
   (d) Not warming it, but offering food and water.

Q8. *Prior to hibernation the tortoise should be:*
   (a) Given a vitamin injection.
   (b) Wormed.
   (c) Offered food up until hibernation.
   (d) None of the above.

Q9. *Animals that require UV light should be:*
   (a) Placed next to a window.
   (b) Placed next to a UV light source.
   (c) Placed next to a UV light source that is changed every 6 months.
   (d) Placed next to a household light bulb.

Q10. *In order to confirm hypocalcaemia:*
   (a) Ionized blood calcium levels should be taken.
   (b) Serum calcium levels should be taken.
   (c) Radiography should be used.
   (d) Urinalysis should be performed.

Answers

Anatomy and physiology
Q1. (a)
Q2. (b)
Q3. (a)
Q4. (c)
Q5. (d)
Q6. (b)
Q7. (d)
Q8. (a)
Q9. (c)
Q10. (b)

Nutrients
Q1. (b)
Q2. (a)
Q3. (b)
Q4. (b)
Q5. (a)
Q6. (c)
Q7. (c)
Q8. (a)
Q9. (a)
Q10. (b)

Feeding calculations
Q1. (d)
Q2. (a)
Q3. (c)
Q4. (a)
Q5. (c)
Q6. (a)
Q7. (d)
Q8. (b)
Q9. (c)
Q10. (d)

Food and feeding
Q1. (d)
Q2. (d)

Q3. (d)
Q4. (a)
Q5. (b)
Q6. (a)
Q7. (b)
Q8. (c)
Q9. (a)
Q10. (d)

Lifestage diets
Q1. (a)
Q2. (b)
Q3. (c)
Q4. (a)
Q5. (d)
Q6. (b)
Q7. (c)
Q8. (b)
Q9. (a)
Q10. (d)

Clinical nutrition
Q1. (a)
Q2. (d)
Q3. (d)
Q4. (b)
Q5. (d)

Q6. (d)
Q7. (a)
Q8. (c)
Q9. (d)
Q10. (d)
Q11. (d)
Q12. (c)
Q13. (d)
Q14. (a)
Q15. (a)
Q16. (d)
Q17. (d)
Q18. (b)
Q19. (d)
Q20. (a)

Exotics
Q1. (c)
Q2. (b)
Q3. (d)
Q4. (d)
Q5. (d)
Q6. (a)
Q7. (b)
Q8. (b)
Q9. (c)
Q10. (a)

Appendix 7
Glossary

Absorption – the uptake of substrates into or across tissues.

Acceptability – a measure of whether a sufficient quantity of a food will be consumed to meet the animal's energy requirements.

Ad libitum feeding – at pleasure or performed with freedom: refers usually to providing an animal with unlimited access to food or water. Can also be referred to as free-choice feeding.

Anabolism – the combination of physical and chemical processes by which living tissue is built up and maintained.

Anorexia – lack or loss of appetite; with complete anorexia the patients will eat nothing, whereas in partial anorexia the patient will eat some food but less than is required to meet resting energy requirement.

Anthropomorphic – attributing human-based perceptions to the pet's needs or preferences.

Antioxidant – 1. a nutrient or non-nutrient substance that prevents formation of free radicals. 2. one of many synthetic or natural substances added to food to prevent or delay its deterioration via oxidation by either combining with free radicals or by scavenging oxygen.

Antivitamin – a factor in the diet that degrades or inhibits a vitamin.

Aromatic amino acids – the amino acids tyrosine, phenylalanine and tryptophan, which are characterized by having a benzene ring.

As-fed basis – concentration of a nutrient in the food as it is fed to an animal; the nutrient concentration is adjusted to include the water content of the food.

Ash – the incombustible inorganic residue remaining after incineration; this is generally the mineral content of the food.

Association of American Feed Control Officials (AAFCO) – agency that develops official pet food regulations of the USA.

Attrition (dental) – excessive wear of the teeth due to tooth-to-tooth contact during mastication.

Atwater values – theoretical gross energy values for protein (4 kcal/g), carbohydrate (4 kcal/g) and fat (9 kcal/g).

Availability (bioavailability) – the degree to which a drug or nutrient becomes available to the target tissue after administration or consumption.

Azotaemia – the presence of an abnormally high concentration of urea, creatinine and other non-protein nitrogenous substances in the blood.

Bacterial translocation – bacteria moving from one place (gut lumen) into another (bloodstream) because of mucosal breakdown.

Balanced food, ration or diet – 1. one that provides an animal with the proper required amounts and proportions of all the nutrients needed for a 24-hour period; avoiding any deficiencies and excesses. 2. all non-energy nutrients in the food are in the correct concentration to the energy density of the food.

Basal energy requirement (BER) – the energy requirement for normal animals in a thermoneutral environment, awake but not moving (resting), and in a post-absorptive state.

Body condition score (BCS) – an assessment of an animal's relative proportions, using both visual assessments and palpation, and comparing the animal under examination with a stereotyped animal on a chart.

Borborygmus – rumbling noise produced by movement of gas through the bowel.

Branched-chain amino acid – the amino acids isoleucine, valine and leucine, which are characterized structurally as having an alkyl side chain, each with a methyl group branch.

Cachexia – a profound state of general ill health and starvation, characterized by severe body wasting.

Caecotroph or caecotrope – a specialized faecal pellet produced in the caecum of rabbits and some rodents. Ingestion of the caecotrophs is termed caecotrophy.

Calculolytic food – a food that produces oversaturation of the urine with calculogenic materials (those that form uroliths).

Catabolic/catabolism – the phase of cellular metabolism where complex nutrient substances are degraded in steps into simpler, smaller end-products.

Cholangiohepatitis – inflammation of the biliary ducts and liver.

Cholangitis – inflammation of the biliary ducts.

Cholestasis – suppression or stoppage of bile flow. This can be due to intrahepatic pressure or extrahepatic causes.

Chyle – an emulsion of lymph and triglycerides absorbed into the lacteals from the GIT lumen during digestion.

Chylomicron – the collection of triglyceride fats together with small amounts of phospholipids and protein absorbed into the lacteals.

Colitis – inflammation of the colon.

Conjugated protein – a protein united with a non-protein molecule.

Cystitis – inflammation of the bladder.

Daily energy requirement (DER) – the total daily energy requirement of an animal. This is normally calculated by multiplying the resting energy requirement by a factor that represents the specifics of that individual animal, e.g. age, activity level, etc.

Diarrhoea – the abnormal increase in frequency, volume or fluidity of faeces, resulting from an overall increase in the water content of the stool.

Diastema – the space in the dental arch between the incisors and canines and cheek teeth, seen in horses, rabbits and some rodents. Can be referred to as the interdental space.

Dietetic – dietetic pet food is the term used in Europe to describe pet foods sold by veterinary practices for the management or prevention of specific conditions.

Dry matter basis – an expression of the nutrient content of food or the requirements of an animal on a moisture-free basis.

Eicosanoid(s) – a group of compounds that are derived from arachidonic acid (e.g. prostaglandins and leukotrienes).

Energy basis – concentration of a nutrient in food expressed as unit of energy, usually per 100 kcal of metabolizable energy.

Energy density – the concentration of energy in a particular food or nutrient.

Enteral feeding – the use of the upper digestive tract (mouth, oesophagus, stomach and small intestine) as the route for assisted feeding.

Fermentation – the anaerobic enzymatic conversion of organic compounds to simpler compounds, such as carbohydrates to volatile fatty acids/short-chain fatty acids. This is an essential process of digestion in the caecum and colon.

Flatulence – the excessive production of gases in the stomach or intestine.

Food-restricted meal feeding – a method of feeding in which a specific quantity of food is fed at specific times/intervals during the day.

Gastric stasis – a reduction in the motility of the stomach, resulting in retention of the gastric contents.

Gluconeogenesis – the production of glucose from a non-carbohydrate source.

Glucose intolerance – the impaired cellular uptake or metabolism of glucose. This can be caused by certain metabolic or receptor abnormalities, resulting in hyperglycaemia, hyperinsulinaemia and/or abnormal patterns of insulin secretion in response to the specific glucose load.

Glycoaminoglycans – polysaccharides associated with proteins that form an integral part of the interstitial fluid, cartilage, skin and tendons.

Glycogenesis – the conversion of glucose to glycogen for storage in the liver.

Glycogenolysis – the splitting of glycogen to provide glucose, occurring in the liver or muscles of the animal.

Glycolysis – the enzymatic conversion of glucose to lactate or pyruvate, releasing energy.

Gout – deposition of urates around and in the joints of the animal, caused through a disorder of the uric acid metabolism.

Gross energy (GE) – the total potential energy content of a food. The GE is determined through use of a bomb calorimeter.

Guaranteed analysis – found on the food label, which lists or guarantees the specific levels of nutrients within the diet. In the USA minimums and maximums of nutrients are listed.

Heat increment – the heat produced through the digestion and metabolism of food.

Hindgut fermenter – animals that digest and assimilate their food primarily through the process of fermentation in the caecum and large intestine.

Homeostasis – a tendency to keep the internal body (chemically and physiologically) stable, in equilibrium.

Humectant – a substance that adds or retains moisture, commonly used in semi-moist diets, e.g. high-fructose corn syrup, propylene glycol or glycerine.

Hydrolysis – the breaking down of a compound by the addition of water.

Hypermetabolism – increase in metabolism.

Hyperplasia – an abnormal increase in the volume of a tissue or organ due to the formation of new cells.

Hypertrophy – an increase in the volume of a tissue or organ due to enlargement of the pre-existing cells.

Hypothalamus – the part of the brain that regulates endocrine activity, thirst and hunger.

Icterus – yellowing of the mucous membranes or skin. Also referred to as jaundice.

Immunocompetence – the ability to develop an immune response after exposure to an antigen.

Ingesta – substances taken to the body via the mouth.

Jejunum – the portion of the small intestine extending from the duodenum to the ileum.

Joule – a measurement of energy. The work done by a force of 1 Newton acting over a distance of 1 metre.

Ketoacidosis – resulting from metabolic acidosis, the accumulation of ketones in the blood. Usually occurring in uncontrolled diabetes mellitus.

Ketone – a metabolic product derived from the catabolism of fatty acids.

Kibble – extruded, formed, individual pieces of dry pet food.

Labial – anatomical term referring to the tooth surface towards the lips.

Lacteal – a capillary of the lymphatic system found within the villus of the small intestine.

Lactose – simple carbohydrate/sugar derived from milk.

Lactulose – a disaccharide that cannot be digested by mammals, but can be fermented in the colon by bacteria into galactose and fructose.

Lean body mass – the portion of the active metabolic body, exclusive of any stored fat.

Learned aversion – avoidance of a particular food by the animal because previous consumption of the food was associated with an unpleasant event (e.g. burned mouth, nausea or rancid foods).

Lingual – anatomical term referring to the mandibular tooth surface towards the tongue.

Lipoprotein – responsible for transporting lipids within the blood, a molecule consisting of both lipid and protein.

Lymphangiectasia – the dilation of the lymphatic vessels.

Maintenance energy requirements (MER) – the energy requirement for an animal in a thermoneutral environment, being moderately active. This energy requirement includes energy required for digestion and absorption of food.

Malabsorption – an impaired intestinal absorption of nutrients from food.

Melaena – presence of digested blood in the faeces, resulting in black tarry stools.

Metabolic water – water in the body that is derived from chemical reactions during the metabolism of nutrients.

Metabolism – the combination of anabolism and catabolism.

Metabolizable energy (ME) – the energy available to the animal once energy from faeces, urine and gases has been removed. Digestible energy minus urinary energy.

Micelle – a sphere formed from bile salts joined with lipids to create a stable, structured fat droplet in water.

National Research Council (NRC) – a private, non-profit organization that evaluates and compiles research work performed by other parties.

Net energy (NE) – the metabolizable energy, minus the heat increment.

Net weight – the declaration of the net quantity of the contents of the food on the packaging. Usually displayed in grams, kilograms, ounces or pounds.

Nutraceutical – a specific nutrient or substance used in the treatment or prevention of a disease. Usually implies the administration of nutrients in amounts that exceed their known dietary requirements.

Obesity – an increase in bodyweight to 20% or more above the animal's optimal weight, due to excessive adipose (fat) tissue.

Obstipation – the passage of watery, soft faeces around a faecal impaction.

Oedema – an abnormal excessive accumulation of fluid within the cavities and intercellular spaces of the body.

Oesophagitis – inflammation of the oesophagus.

Overweight – when the animal weighs between 10-19% more than its optimal weight, due to excessive adipose (fat) tissue.

Palatability – a measure of preference; how much an animal likes a food.

Parenchyma – the functional elements of an organ.

Parenteral – administration of a substance or food via a route other than the alimentary tract.

Pica – craving or eating unusual substances, unnatural articles of food or foreign materials.

Postprandial – the period occurring after meals; can also be referred to as postcibal.

Precipitation – the deposition of solid particles of a substance from a solution.

Regurgitation – a backward flow of ingesta (normally undigested food).

Resorption – reabsorption.

Resting energy requirement (RER) – the energy required by a relaxed animal in a thermoneutral environment 12 hours after eating.

Rugae – folds or ridges, as seen in the stomach.

Satiety – the feeling of having fulfilled all the desires to eat and drink.

Steatorrhoea – the presence of fats in the faeces.

Struvite – type of crystals commonly seen in cats experiencing FLUTD; otherwise known as magnesium-ammonium-phosphate hexahydrate or triple-phosphate crystals.

Supersaturated solution – a solution that has a higher concentration of a substance dissolved within it than would be expected.

Supplement – a concentrated nutrient source that is added to the basic diet.

Table food – foods that are usually consumed by people, but also fed to pets.

Tenesmus – the act of straining to pass urine or faeces.

Time-restricted feeding – a method of feeding where the animal can consume an unlimited quantity of food within a set period of time, usually 5–10 minutes, at specific intervals throughout the day.

Transit time – the time taken for ingested food to pass through the digestive system.

Trichobezoar – a hairball.

Uraemia – an excess of urea and creatinine and other nitrogenous waste products within the blood.

Urethritis – inflammation of the urethra.

Urolith – a calculus in the urine or urinary tract that usually contains more than 90% organic or inorganic crystalloids.

Urolithiasis – the formation of urinary stones within the urinary tract from less-soluble crystalloids in the urine.

Visceral – relating to the intestinal organs of the body.

Vitamin – a general term referring to a number of different unrelated organic substances that are essential in specific amounts for normal metabolism.

Vomiting – the forcible ejection of the stomach contents through the mouth, also referred to as emesis.

Workload – expected work done over a period of time.

Index

W

Y

Z